Vascular Damage in Neglected Tropical Diseases

Valeria Silvestri · Vivian Mushi
Billy Ngasala

Vascular Damage in Neglected Tropical Diseases

A Surgical Perspective

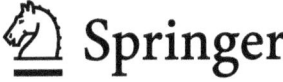 Springer

Valeria Silvestri
Parasitology and Medical Entomology
Muhimbili University of Health and Allied
Sciences
Dar es Salaam, Tanzania

Vivian Mushi
Parasitology and Medical Entomology
Muhimbili University of Health and Allied
Sciences
Dar es Salaam, Tanzania

Billy Ngasala
Parasitology and Medical Entomology
Muhimbili University of Health and Allied
Sciences
Dar es Salaam, Tanzania

ISBN 978-3-031-53352-5   ISBN 978-3-031-53353-2   (eBook)
https://doi.org/10.1007/978-3-031-53353-2

This Springer imprint is published by the registered company Springer Nature Switzerland AG
The registered company address is: Gewerbestrasse 11, 6330 Cham, Switzerland

If disposing of this product, please recycle the paper.

Contents

Contents

Introduction

Neglected Tropical Disease: Definition

Neglected tropical diseases were first mentioned as such in the early 2000s, as a group of health disorders highlighted within the Millennium Development Goal. These conditions shared common features, including the fact of being chronic and debilitating infections, in many cases of parasitic aetiology, which mostly occurred among the extreme poor [1]. The phrase "neglected" indicates that they were eclipsed by other diseases such as HIV, tuberculosis and malaria [2].

According to the updated and actual WHO definition, neglected tropical diseases (NTDs) are a diverse group of 20 conditions mainly prevalent in tropical areas, where they affect more than 1 billion people who live in impoverished communities [3]. Specifically, the list includes: Buruli ulcer, Chagas disease, dengue, and chikungunya, dracunculiasis (Guinea-worm disease), echinococcosis, foodborne trematodiases, human African trypanosomiasis (sleeping sickness), leishmaniasis, leprosy

(Hansen's disease), lymphatic filariasis, mycetoma, chromoblastomycosis and other deep mycoses, onchocerciasis (river blindness), podoconiosis, rabies, scabies and other ectoparasitoses, schistosomiasis, soil-transmitted helminthiases, snakebite envenoming, taeniasis/cysticercosis, trachoma, yaws and other endemic treponematoses [4].

The devastating health consequences that characterize each condition usually overlap huge socioeconomic consequences that are due to the reduction of population productivity and are increased by the lack of access to quality healthcare. The marginalization of those populations living in endemic settings, a lack of funding for healthcare systems and inadequate data on disease prevalence and control are also great contributors to the diseases' neglect, making them a public health challenge [2].

Neglected Tropical Diseases: General Epidemiology

The interest in tropical diseases started during the nineteenth century, with the establishment of tropical institutes in countries with large colonial holdings. Only later, the definition of tropical illnesses was integrated with the term "neglected", to better define those conditions affecting populations from resource-poor countries in tropical and sub-tropical regions [5, 6]. People living in these settings experience an inadequate access to safe sanitation, to safe water supply and to government health centres [7]. In this sense, NTDs' epidemiology reflects those health inequities which are main drivers of the NTD burden and shows higher prevalence of these conditions in developing countries compared to developed ones [2]. The global burden of NTDs is reported in the WHO's roadmap 2021–2030, which is available at https://www.who.int/publications/i/item/9789240010352 and reported in Fig. 1.1.

The African Setting

Africa accounts for about 40% of the global burden of NTDs, with about 600 million individuals requiring treatment. At least one NTD is endemic in each country in the African region, and 79% of African countries are co-endemic with at least five of them [2]. Schistosomiasis, lymphatic filariasis and onchocerciasis emerge among the great challenges. The continent accounts for up to 90% of schistosomiasis cases, with 280,000 deaths estimated yearly due to this parasitosis. For lymphatic filariasis and onchocerciasis, the estimated at-risk population in Africa requiring intervention was 341 and 220 million people, respectively [2, 8].

The Asian Setting

Analysing the Asian setting, it was observed that the first five helminth infections in the WHO list, specifically soil-transmitted helminthiases, schistosomiasis, foodborne trematodiases, lymphatic filariasis and taeniasis/cysticercosis, are still endemic. These infections are mainly reported from eastern Asian countries, where almost 200 million people, mostly indigenous, face extreme poverty, specifically in Indonesia, the Philippines, Myanmar, Viet Nam and Cambodia and among upper

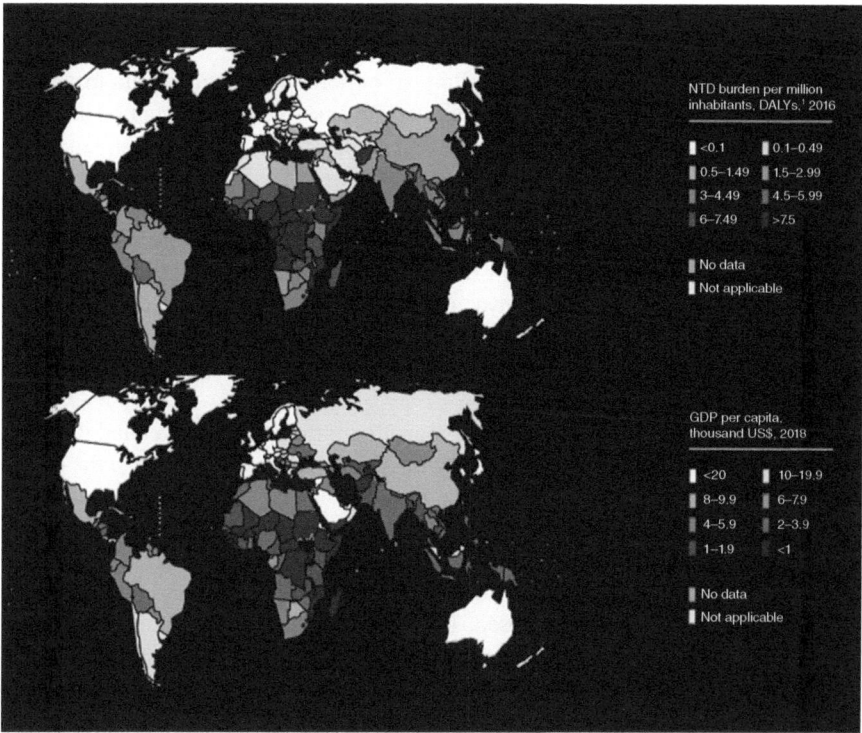

Fig. 1.1 Geographical spread of the NTD burden, by DALY and gross domestic product. Figure from the WHO's document Ending the neglect to attain the Sustainable Development Goals: A road map for neglected tropical diseases 2021–2030 (who.int) [3]

middle-income countries such as Malaysia and Thailand. As described in the African setting, in Asia, schistosomiasis and lymphatic filariasis are among the most common NTDs, and each helminthiasis is associated with approximately 100 million infections in the region. In addition, more than 10 million people suffer from either liver or intestinal fluke infections, as well as schistosomiasis and lymphatic filariasis [9]. Current conditions and developments in Asia will sustain what was defined as "the yin and yang" of NTDs. In other words, while the reduction of poverty and effective control activities will work towards the decline of NTDs, other factors as urbanization, food insecurity and environmental and climate change will contribute to the persistence of distinct NTDs [9].

The Latin America Setting

Since the start of the twenty-first century, Latin America faced socio-political and economic challenges due to prolonged droughts, intermittent and extreme floods due to climate change, drug trade, food insecurity from agricultural declines, human displacements, urbanization and the marginalization of large indigenous populations. All these factors have shaped the epidemiological scenario of NTD in Latin

America, reducing the public health gains regarding the NTDs in this continent, making this region a global "hotspot" for NTDs [10].

The decline in health systems resulting from political and economic instability likely accounts for the scarce public health achievements in the prevention and control of NTD in this vulnerable setting. Additionally, because of Central America's vulnerability to climate change, the recent formation of a dry corridor in central regions can also promote the susceptibility of this region to vector-borne tropical diseases. This adds to the interruption of vector control activities, which has been detrimental, leading to a significant rise in Chagas disease, leishmaniasis, dengue and the emergence of chikungunya and *Zika virus* infections. Schistosomiasis increases have also been noted in endemic hotspots [10].

Non-Endemic Setting

In recent years, factors such as climate change, migrations and travel and the presence of local conflicts in the endemic regions can additionally challenge the epidemiological context of NTDs by moving diseases outside the limit of the endemic regions of the tropical belt. As a result, these diseases can now be more frequently diagnosed in industrialized countries with temperate climates [5–7].

Because most NTDs do not require hospitalization and several cases of illegal migrants might remain undiagnosed, the prevalence of these conditions in non-endemic countries might be underestimated [5]. This fact emphasizes the importance of increasing global awareness of NTDs among healthcare professionals to improve clinical management and control of such diseases also in non-endemic settings [5].

Prevention and Control Strategies. The Need for Morbidity Management

To address this specific global health issue, WHO set the first NTD road map (2012–2020) [4]. According to it, NTDs are approached through five strategies: preventive chemotherapy, intensified disease management, vector control, veterinary public health measures for zoonotic neglected diseases and improved water and sanitation [6]. A vertical approach through massive drug administration (MDA), the distribution of preventive chemotherapy during prevention and control campaigns, is central to WHO's prevention and control strategy for many NTDs [7].

As a result of the implementation of the prescriptions of the first road map, the population requiring NTD interventions decreased by 25% between 2010 and 2021, from 2.19 to 1.65 billion. As of the end of 2022, 47 countries have eliminated at least one NTD; more than 1 billion people were treated for at least one NTD each year from 2015 through to 2019 [4].

Still, notwithstanding interventions in place, the burden of NTDs continues to have an unequal global impact, with 80% of this burden affecting 16 countries. The progress in high-burden countries was slower than expected and uneven across certain of the 20 diseases and disease groups, while persistent risk factors such as poverty, climate change and rapid population growth emerge as threats to achieving the 2030 targets within the defined timescales [11].

Additionally, the dominant vertical approach to the prevention and control of NTDs showed some limits.

One of the major concerns related to the vertical approach to NTDs is the unavailability of drugs donated for prevention and control of these conditions in healthcare centres for clinical practice use outside the setting of the intervention campaigns, thus leaving untreated the infected patients that are not the target of the distribution [12]. Additionally, chronic conditions can go well beyond the active infection, and the public health impact of NTDs is not limited to mortality, but can extend to disability and morbidity [7, 13]. Because of the primary focus of NTD policy on disease elimination, chronic NTDs and their associated morbidity impact have only recently been recognized [14]. These concepts were well described and emphasized in a comprehensive paper by Chami et al., which focused on how a vertical approach is sub-optimal to address all issues related to NTDs because it can't guarantee equitable access to treatment nor comprehensively address morbidity issues outside the prevention and control goal [7].

The need for chronic morbidity management in NTDs urgently calls for a new comprehensive strategy, combining MDA with on-demand access to treatment within local health systems [7]. This new perspective moves from the disease-specific management to a cross-cutting approach of coordinated and multi-disciplinary NTD programmes that could finally be integrated into national health systems [6, 15].

In this sense, the new roadmap for 2021–2030 sets out key actions and programmatic shifts to drive progress towards a world free of NTDs by 2030 [4] and supports the vision of universal health coverage, in which all individuals and communities receive the health services they need without suffering financial hardship [3]. Among the 2030 targets and milestones, special importance is given to disease control, in terms of reduction to locally acceptable levels not only of the incidence and prevalence but also of their morbidity and/or mortality [3].

Different targets have been set to define a successful disease control, according to different diseases. For some of the conditions included in this text, as in the case for filariasis, the goal is to eliminate the condition as a public health threat, with the infection sustained below the thresholds of transmission for at least 4 years after stopping mass drug administration, together with the availability of an essential package of care for patients affected by morbidity due to previous infection sequelae. Different parameters are considered for schistosomiasis: the elimination as a public health problem is currently defined as <1% proportion of heavy-intensity schistosomiasis infections [3]. For other conditions, the goal includes intensifying control (such as in the case of echinococcosis in hyperendemic areas); the incorporation of management in the universal health coverage package of care, as in the case for ectoparasites as scabies, or the reduction of mortality by 50%, as for the neglected frequently fatal snakebite envenomation [3].

Independently from the specific target set for disease control, a better understanding of disease epidemiology and pathology, together with the availability of effective diagnostic tools (that can reduce progression to severe morbidity and disability by ensuring early detection and management), and the availability of effective, affordable interventions for prevention, case management, treatment and rehabilitation are constantly at the core of the new roadmap [3], through the promotion of cross-sectoral collaboration centred on the needs of people and communities, including issues of stigma and disability [16]. Capacity planning is also emerging as central to ensure affordable access to surgery and management of complications [3].

In this new way of conceiving disease and related chronic comorbidities and disabilities, an exhaustive comprehension of the pathophysiology behind each specific condition is essential, including the ones addressed in this book.

Vascular Damage in Patients with NTDs: A General View

The burden and public health impact of many NTDs are not limited to the acute phase of the infection or to it related mortality, but extend to chronic sequelae that lead to morbidity and permanent disability. In this sense, non-communicable manifestations such as damage of cardiovascular or cerebrovascular interest or oncologic lesions are to be considered as part of the NTD burden [17–20].

Previous studies described several mechanisms of vascular damage of surgical interest in patients with different NTDs. Many of these mechanisms, such as endothelial damage, vasa vasorum arteritis or induction of atherosclerosis damage [21, 22], are shared by other infectious conditions that are known to be associated with vascular lesions, (for example, tertiary syphilis or HIV), while other mechanisms are specific of each condition.

In this book, we will analyse in detail the vascular damage of surgical interest occurring in patients affected by different NTDs, which we can briefly summarizes as follows.

Vascular complications in schistosomiasis can be caused by haemodynamic impairment, secondary to the chronic granulomatous inflammation of embolized eggs reaching the arteriolar districts of perfused organs, through direct damage to the arterial wall or through additional mechanisms, including vasa vasorum obliterative endarteritis, direct endothelium damage or the induction of atherosclerotic degeneration [20]. These mechanisms can lead to aneurysm lesions, vasculitis with or without vascular stenosis or stroke [17, 20].

In patients with echinococcosis, arterial damage can be secondary to a primary hydatid intramural form, to the spontaneous or surgical rupture of a hydatid cyst into an adjacent vessel, to the erosion of the arterial wall of the aorta from adjacent organs or vertebral lesions, by scolex passing into the vasa vasorum through an intimal defect [17, 18].

Amoebiasis, a globally endemic protozoal infection causing a range of gastroenteric manifestations or extra-enteric involvement, is not included in the list of NTD recognized by WHO, but it has been considered for this book in the perspective of an expanded definition of these diseases [1]. Vascular lesions in amoebiasis are described occasionally as extra-intestinal manifestations of the infection, specifically in the hepatic vessels, on which a direct action of trophozoites on the hepatic vascular wall was suggested [23].

In the case of lymphatic filariasis, a filarial helminthiasis known to affect lymphatic vessels, the vascular damage can occur in the chronic phase of the infection as oncologic vascular lesions, in the form of lymphangiosarcoma. Oncogenesis, in this case, could be favoured by lymph stasis, which impairs immune cell migration, local immune response and angiogenesis [24]. Malignant transformation of the endothelium can eventually occur and develop on this induced microenvironment [25].

Ectoparasites are not spared from being involved in vascular damage, and reports are available for kind of infestation. It is the case for tungiasis, caused by *Tunga penetrans* infection. Diabetic patients are at risk of developing foot ulcers, as a result of many factors including hyperglycaemia, trauma, underlying diabetic peripheral neuropathy and peripheral arterial disease [26]. In cases where diabetes is complicated by peripheral neuropathy and vascular impairment, *T. penetrans* infection and trauma following its extraction may predispose to rapidly progressing ulcer, with potentially unfavourable outcomes due to sepsis and death [26].

Finally, among non-parasitic NTDs, vascular complications are described for snakebite envenomation. Lesions may occur from days to weeks after envenomation, due to enzymatic components of venom or mechanical injury at the bite site [27]. Damage can occur in the absence of local effects [27], likely due to intra-arterial injection of the venom through wall penetration [27] or because of the local action of the venom injected in proximity of the involved artery [27, 28]. Proteolytic enzymes contained in venom can destroy the structural components of the arterial wall or its extracellular matrix; through direct endothelial damage, with the induction of apoptosis in endothelial cells [27, 29]; through the necrosis of arterial wall and surrounding tissues [28] or through the inflammatory mechanisms mediated by reactive oxygen species and cytokines [27].

A summary of the pathophysiology mechanisms linking NTDs to vascular damage is provided in Fig. 1.2.

Challenges in Addressing Vascular Lesions in NTDs

Cardiovascular or neurovascular complications of surgical interest that affect patients with NTDs can be considered as non-communicable complications that derive from these conditions. Because vascular damage in patients affected by these conditions could follow different patterns from the classic atherosclerosis, the understanding of the pathophysiology behind vascular lesions in patients affected by NTDs, of their clinical manifestations and of their natural course is urgently needed. This knowledge will constitute an essential tool to target comorbidity management, in addition to prevention and control interventions aiming at lowering and interrupting disease transmission, as included in the new WHO roadmap [3].

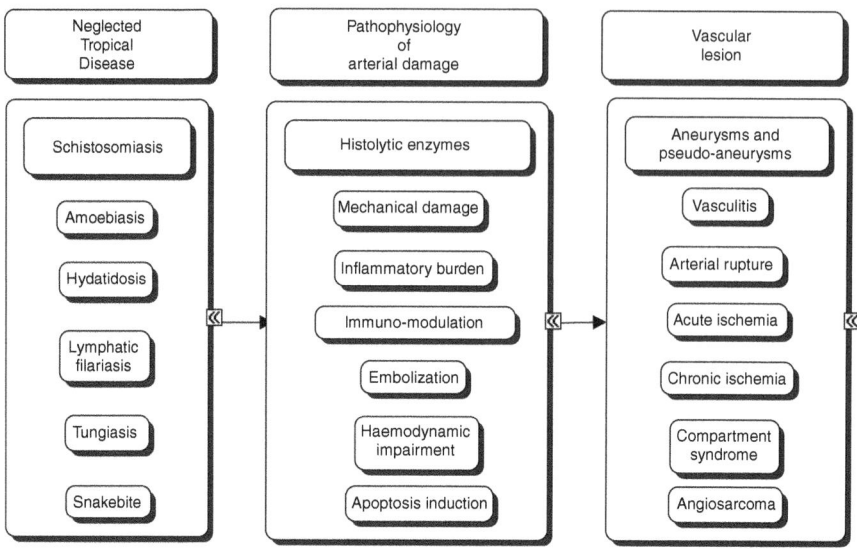

Fig. 1.2 From NTDs to vascular lesions. A schematic view

Independently from their aetiology, non-communicable diseases (NCDs) represent a major public health concern globally, rapidly increasing in prevalence in low- and middle-income countries (LMICs). The World Health Organization estimated that, taken together, NCDs are responsible for 71% of the world's death yearly and accountable for 41 million deaths yearly. The highest burden is expected in LMICs, where most of the NCDs deaths (74%) and the majority of premature deaths (86%) occur. It was estimated that in 2030, around 80% of those deaths will come from LMICs, predicting about 52 million deaths yearly.

When tackling the issue of NDCs in LMICs, there are challenges related to this specific setting to consider, mainly the insufficient availability of quality diagnostic tools; barriers to access of quality surgery; challenges in the research system, including the lack of available data. It is important to consider this peculiar scenario, to better understand why we know so little on the topic of vascular diseases in these settings and to conceive the challenges and barriers to be overcome when planning to fill these gaps.

To tackle the issue of non-communicable disease (including surgical vascular complications of NTD) in low-income settings, there is a need to define methods for their early detection and diagnoses using low-cost technologies, to allow the effective delivery of these diagnostic interventions and to reduce medical costs for their management, in order to improve the quality of life among affected populations [30]. Previous studies have emphasized the sub-optimal availability of basic technologies, including diagnostic tests and equipment for NCDs, leading to a lack of basic NCD interventions in LMICs. This lack of basic technologies could be a consequence of global fiscal restraint, in those countries that notwithstanding being highly burdened by NCDs, decrease expenditures on social sectors, including health. Enhancing access to essential medicines and basic technologies is crucial for the accomplishment of the Millennium Development Goals [30].

From the perspective of the diagnosis and management of surgical vascular lesions in NTDs, the unavailability of these essential technologies for diagnosis is the first barrier to the clinical observation and definition of these conditions. But it is not the only one.

When we focus our observation on non-communicable complications of surgical interest, we have to keep in mind the issues that surgery as a discipline faces in LMICs. Even though surgery has been increasingly recognized as key to enhancing global health and achieving the Sustainable Development Goals, large gaps exist in global surgical care, including deficiencies in surgical infrastructure, human resources, financing and education occurring in low- and middle-income countries [31]. These gaps translate into challenges in accessibility to surgical care and, importantly, to quality surgical care. Globally, 5 billion people lack access to safe surgical care with more deaths due to lack of quality care rather than lack of access. Even though many proven quality improvement interventions exist in high-income countries, implementing them in low/middle-income countries (LMICs) faces further challenges [30]. In LMICs, the awareness of both clinicians and politicians of promising interventions doesn't directly translate into the ability to implement them, due to challenges that include limited time, resources and the shortage of professional skills [30].

Evidence of vascular damage in patients with NTD is limited to scattered case reports and case series [17, 18, 20, 23]. Given the non-negligible prevalence and burden of the single conditions in endemic areas, it can be hypothesized that reports of occurring vascular co-morbidities could be underestimated.

Factors that characterize the research in endemic areas could strengthen this suggestion of report bias. The developing countries bear the greatest share of the global burden of disease, much of it in tropical settings [32]. Still, research in endemic nations is challenged by multiple factors that lead to a low local capacity to identify and address the root causes of health outcomes, such as chronic underinvestment in universities and research institutions and shortages in well-trained and skilled researchers [33] when compared with local needs.

One of the major issues in describing the epidemiology of health conditions in endemic settings is the lack of exhaustive and reliable data, an essential tool for the improvement of population health and health systems [34]. Access to reliable disease data archives in low- and middle-income countries is one of the major challenges that affect the ability to address unique clinical problems related to these settings and limits global researchers' ability to learn from diverse populations [34]. Despite the introduction of electronic health data systems in low- and middle-income countries (LMICs) to improve the availability, quantity and quality of data, recent studies denounce that some LMICs still have little or no system to efficiently collect and analyse information, and researchers have reported technical challenges due to limitation of data collection forms that prevent the archiving of diseases state. The development of archives for the storage of retrospective data sets is an essential tool for improvement of population health and health systems.

For researchers looking to understand the underlying causes of diseases and create novel therapies and preventive measures, medical data archives can be a significant source of data. The development of new policies and programmes can benefit from this as it can increase our understanding of diseases from a scientific perspective. Additionally, by offering information about the impact of disease on various communities, data allow more precise resource allocation to areas where it is most required [34]. These data sets would be essential also to understand the prevalence, clinical presentation, natural history and outcome of specific comorbidities related to NTD, which up until now have been described only in occasional case reports or series. Retrospective database could expand the number and quality of observations needed to define the hypothesis, guiding future research in unexplored patterns.

Aim of This Book

This book aims to collect and summarize evidence related to vascular complications of surgical interest in specific NTDs, in terms of epidemiology, physiopathology and description of cases, challenges and future perspectives for research. This will provide a state-of-the-art description of the morbidity of vascular surgical interest in patients affected by each condition, addressed in separate chapters. This description of the state of art will be a starting point that could stimulate further discussion and studies on this understudied matter of global urgency.

References

1. Hotez PJ, Aksoy S, Brindley PJ, Kamhawi S. What constitutes a neglected tropical disease? PLoS Negl Trop Dis. 2020;14(1):1–6.
2. George NS, David SC, Nabiryo M, Sunday BA, Olanrewaju OF, Yangaza Y, et al. Addressing neglected tropical diseases in Africa: a health equity perspective. Glob Heal Res Policy. 2023;8(1):30. https://doi.org/10.1186/s41256-023-00314-1.
3. WHO. Ending the neglect to attain the sustainable development goals: a road map for neglected tropical diseases 2021–2030. Geneva: WHO; 2020. 196 p.
4. WHO. Neglected Tropical Diseases. 2023. Available from: https://www.who.int/news-room/questions-and-answers/item/neglected-tropical-diseases.
5. Casulli A, Antinori S, Bartoloni A, D'Amelio S, Gabrielli AF, Gazzoli G, et al. Neglected tropical diseases in Italy: introducing IN-NTD, the Italian network for NTDs. Parasitology. 2023;150(12):1082–8.
6. Molyneux DH, Savioli L, Engels D. Neglected tropical diseases: progress towards addressing the chronic pandemic. Lancet. 2017;389(10066):312–25.
7. Chami GF, Bundy DAP. More medicines alone cannot ensure the treatment of neglected tropical diseases. Lancet Infect Dis. 2019;19(9):e330–6.
8. WHO. Onchocerciasis. 2022. Available from: https://www.who.int/news-room/fact-sheets/detail/onchocerciasis.
9. Sripa B, Leonardo L, Hong SJ, Ito A, Brattig NW. Status and perspective of asian neglected tropical diseases, 106212. Acta Trop. 2022;225 https://doi.org/10.1016/j.actatropica.2021.106212.
10. Hotez PJ, Damania A, Bottazzi ME. Central Latin America: two decades of challenges in neglected tropical disease control. PLoS Negl Trop Dis. 2020;14(3):1–7. https://doi.org/10.1371/journal.pntd.0007962.

11. WHO. Global report on neglected tropical diseases 2023: Executive summary. World Heal Organ; 2023. Available from: https://www.who.int/publications/i/item/9789240069015.

12. Zacharia F, Silvestri V, Mushi V, Ogweno G, Makene T, Mhamilawa LE. Burden and factors associated with ongoing transmission of soil-transmitted helminths infections among the adult population: a community-based cross-sectional survey in Muleba district, Tanzania. PLoS One. 2023;18(7):e0288936. https://doi.org/10.1371/journal.pone.0288936.

13. Van't Noordende AT, Kuiper H, Ramos AN, Mieras LF, Barbosa JC, SMF P, et al. Towards a toolkit for cross-neglected tropical disease morbidity and disability assessment. Int Health. 2015;8(Suppl 1):i71–81.

14. Bailey F, Eaton J, Jidda M, van Brakel WH, Addiss DG, Molyneux DH. Neglected tropical diseases and mental health: Progress, partnerships, and integration. Trends Parasitol. 2019;35(1):23–31. https://doi.org/10.1016/j.pt.2018.11.001.

15. Lancet T. Neglected tropical diseases: ending the neglect of populations. Lancet. 2022;399(10323):411.

16. Addiss DG, Kienast Y, Lavery JV. Ethical dimensions of neglected tropical disease programming. Trans R Soc Trop Med Hyg. 2021;115(2):190–5.

17. Silvestri V, Mushi V, Ngasala B, Kihwele J, Sabas D, Rocchi L. Stroke in patients with schistosomiasis: review of cases in literature. Can J Infect Dis Med Microbiol. 2022;2022:3902570.

18. Silvestri V, Mushi V, Mshana MI, Bonaventure WM, Justine N, Kihwele J, et al. Aortic aneurysm lesions in echinococcus infection. A review of cases in literature, vol. 50. Travel Medicine and Infectious Disease. Elsevier Ltd; 2022. p. 102476.

19. Silvestri V, Mshana MI, Mushi V, Bonaventura WM, Justine NC, Kinabo C, et al. Subclinical vascular damage in Schistosoma spp. endemic regions: a community based cross-sectional study in Kome Island, Tanzania. Vasa Eur J Vasc Med. 2023:1–9.

20. Silvestri V, Mushi V, Mshana MI, Bonaventura WM, Justine NC, Sabas D, et al. Blood flukes and arterial damage: a review of aneurysm cases in patients with schistosomiasis. Can J Infect Dis Med Microbiol. 2022;2022:6483819.

21. De Rango P, De Socio GV, Silvestri V, Simonte G, Verzini F. An unusual case of epigastric and back pain expanding descending thoracic aneurysm resulting from tertiary syphilis diagnosed with positron emission tomography. Circ Cardiovasc Imaging. 2013;6:1120–1.

22. Silvestri V, D'Ettorre G, Borrazzo C, Mele R. Many different patterns under a common flag: aortic pathology in HIV. Review of case reports in literature. Ann Vasc Surg. 2019;8(59):268–84.

23. Silvestri V, Ngasala B. Hepatic aneurysm in patients with amoebic liver abscess. A review of cases in literature, 102274. Travel Med Infect Dis. 2022;46 https://doi.org/10.1016/j.tmaid.2022.102274.

24. Walke VA, Datar S, Kowe B, Chaurasia JK. Unusual coexistence of Stewart-Treves syndrome and sickle cell anaemia: a case of dual pathology. BMJ Case Rep. 2022;15(7):1–4.

25. Krishnamoorthy N, Viswanathan S, Rekhi B, Jambhekar NA. Lymphangiosarcoma arising after 33 years within a background of chronic filariasis: a case report with review of literature. J Cutan Pathol. 2012;39(1):52–5.

26. Ebrahim AA, Mpango EP, Temba JA, Abbas ZG, Mashili FL. Tunga penetrans causing a rapidly progressing foot ulcer in a patient with uncontrolled type 2 diabetes mellitus. Oxford Med Case Rep. 2022;2(3):85–8.

27. Russell C, Senthilkumaran S, Miller SW, Williams HF, Vaiyapuri R, Savania R, et al. Ultrasound-guided compression method effectively counteracts Russell's viper bite-induced pseudoaneurysm. Toxins. 2022;14(4):4–11.

28. Linfeng W, Lutao X, Pin L, Linjie L, Meisong C, Wang D. Toxicon radial artery aneurysm formation and spontaneous rupture after snake bite to the right forearm. Toxicon. 2020;181(April):79–81.

29. Senthilkumaran S, Miller SW, Williams HF, Savania R, Thirumalaikolundusubramanian P, Patel K, et al. Toxicon development of Wunderlich syndrome following a Russell's viper bite. Toxicon. 2022;215(May):11–6.

30. Albelbeisi AH, Albelbeisi A, El Bilbeisi AH, Taleb M, Takian A, Akbari-Sari A. Public sector capacity to prevent and control of noncommunicable diseases in twelve low- and middle-income countries based on WHO-PEN standards: a systematic review. Heal Serv Insights. 2021;14:1178632920986233.
31. Alayande BT, Hughes Z, Fitzgerald TN, Riviello R, Bekele A, Rice HE. With equity in mind: evaluating an interactive hybrid global surgery course for cross-site interdisciplinary learners. PLOS Glob Public Heal. 2023;3(5):e0001778. https://doi.org/10.1371/journal.pgph.0001778.
32. Kitua AY, Corrah T, Herbst K, Nyirenda T, Agwale S, Makanga M, et al. Strengthening capacity, collaboration and quality of clinical research in Africa: EDCTP Networks of Excellence. Tanzan J Health Res. 2009;11(1):51–4.
33. Izugbara CO, Kabiru CW, Amendah D, Dimbuene ZT, Donfouet HPP, Atake EH, et al. "It takes more than a fellowship program": reflections on capacity strengthening for health systems research in sub-Saharan Africa. BMC Health Serv Res. 2017;17(Suppl 2):1–5.
34. Abdul-rahman T, Ghosh S, Lukman L, Bamigbade GB, Oladipo OV, Amarachi OR, et al. Income countries: mystery behind public health statistics and measures. J Infect Public Health. 2023;16(10):1556–61. https://doi.org/10.1016/j.jiph.2023.07.001.

Schistosomiasis

2

Contents

Introduction

Schistosomiasis: Historical Notes

Schistosomiasis is an infection caused by trematode worms of the genus *Schistosoma* which have different geographical distribution [1, 2]: *Schistosoma haematobium* is endemic in sub-Saharan Africa and Middle East, *Schistosoma mansoni* in sub-Saharan Africa, South America and Caribbeans and *Schistosoma japonicum* is endemic in People's Republic of China, the Philippines and Indonesia [1].

    The first description of cases related to the most prevalent species, *S. haematobium* and *S. mansoni*, were respectively attributed to Theodor Bilharz and Patrick Manson. Urinary schistosomiasis, or Bilharziasis, was named after Theodore Bilharz

(1825–1852), German parasitologist in service in Egypt at the medical school in Cairo, who discovered a flat non-segmented worm in the urinary plexus of a patient assessed for haematuria [3], while in 1902, Sir Patrick Manson, the "Father of Tropical Medicine", reported a case of intestinal schistosomiasis in the stool of a "38-year-old Englishman" [4]. Sir Manson was also the first to consider the existence of an intermediate host for the life cycle of schistosomiasis. This hypothesis was finally confirmed by Robert Thomson Leiper, who understood the complete cycle of *Schistosoma* spp., with the recognition of aquatic snails as intermediate hosts of these trematodes [4].

Thanks to paleopathology studies, we know that *Schistosoma* spp. is affecting humans since antiquity: the most ancient evidence of this parasitic infestation dates back to more than 6000 years ago. Spined *Schistosoma* from the pelvic sediment of human skeletal remains were found in the area of Tell Zeidan, an early settlement of farmers in northern Syria (5800–4000 years before Christ) [4]. Schistosomiasis may have then spread to Egypt as a result of the importation of monkeys and slaves during the reign of the fifth dynasty of pharaohs (~2494–2345 BC) [4]. *S. haematobium* eggs and bladder calcifications were discovered on Egyptian mummies of the XX dynasty by Marc Armand Ruffer (1859–1917), pioneer of paleopathology. This discovery was followed in 1977 by the description of calcified *Schistosome* eggs in the kidney, liver and intestine of Nakht, a mummy 1200 B.C, by a Canadian team [3]. Not limited to Egypt, paleo-pathology studies by Wei in 1973 have reported eggs with *Schistosome* features from China, in a female mummy from the Mawangdui tomb dating back to the Han dynasty (206/202 BC–AD 220) [5]. As for the New World, it was Manson, who, after diagnosing with schistosomiasis an English man who lived in the Caribbean region, suggested that the infection could have been transported to this continent during the times of slavery from Africa [4].

Not only biological reports on human remains but also written documents retrieved by archaeologists suggest that the disease must have been already endemic and of public health importance among populations in the antiquity. Ancient medical documents as Egyptian medical papyri from Egypt (both Ebers and Berlin) describe haematuria as a symptom and suggest remedies for it [3]. The "$\bar{a} - a - \bar{a}$ *disease*", a conditions characterized by discharge from penis, was interpreted as a possible ancient name for schistosomiasis; this symptom is mentioned 22 times in Egyptian medical papyri from as early as 1500 years BC, and this repetition suggests that it was a frequent condition at that time [4].

Epidemiology

Schistosomiasis is an infection caused by one of the five species of trematode worms in the genus *Schistosoma* [1]. The most important species involved in human pathology are *S. haematobium*, responsible for urogenital disease and endemic in Africa and Middle east; *S. mansoni*, endemic in Africa, Middle East, Central and South America and *S. japonicum* endemic in eastern Asia. *S. mansoni* and *S. japonicum* are both responsible for intestinal/hepatic disease) [4]. It affects 250 million people worldwide, 201.5 million in Africa [6], where 90% of infected population live [7]. It is also endemic in parts of Latin America and Asia [7]. The global burden of the disease is of 1.9 million disability-adjusted life years [1].

Recently, increased population movements due to climate changes were directly linked to the spread of Schistosomiasis [1, 8, 9], and autochthonous cases were reported in Corsica, France and Almeria, South-East Spain [7]. Europe receives a constant flow of migrants, among them, a significant proportion comes from schistosomiasis endemic countries. As a consequence of increased migration and travels from endemic settings, the number of people in Europe at risk of having chronic schistosomiasis is becoming potentially high. According to recent data, nearly 24% of SSA migrants test positive for anti-*Schistosoma* spp. sero-assays. Additionally, the diagnosis of schistosomiasis is not unusual among travellers [7].

Pathophysiology and Clinical Manifestations of Schistosomiasis

There are five main pathogenic species of *Schistosoma* spp. that affect humans: *S. mansoni, S. japonicum, S. intercalatum, S. guineensis* and *S. mekongi* and *S. haematobium* [7]. While the adult form of the parasite dwells in human venous plexus, *Schistosoma* spp. life cycle requires a phase of asexual multiplication within an intermediate host, represented by a snail (*Biomphalaria* spp. snails for *S. mansoni, Bulinus* spp. snails for *S. haematobium* and *Oncomelania* spp. snails for *S. japonicum* [1].

Infection in humans occurs through contact with fresh water infested by free-swimming cercariae, released by intermediate host snails, which penetrate intact skin and gain access to venous and lymphatic vessels [10, 11]. The symptomatic stage of the infection occurs 2 weeks to 3 months after exposure, with fever caused by systemic hypersensitivity to schistosomula migration [1]. This stage is followed by an established active infection in which adults lay eggs in blood vessels. Eggs migrate into the intestinal lumen or into the bladder cavity, from where they are released in the environment though stool or urine, but occasionally can remain trapped in the surrounding tissue, leading to granuloma formation and organ damage at entrapment sites. Granuloma formation can cause chronic hepatopathies, liver fibrosis and core-pulmonary disease [9].

S. mansoni, S. japonicum, S. intercalatum, S. guineensis and *S. mekongi* usually cause hepato-intestinal schistosomiasis, while *S. haematobium* affects the urogenital tract [7], but the relation between organs and apparatus involved and *Schistosoma* species is not so strict: ectopic oviposition can occur, explained by the existence of numerous anastomoses of portal vein circulation with veins draining the internal genital organs [12].

In hepato-splenic schistosomiasis, eggs of *S. japonicum* or *S. mansoni* are oviposed from the mesenteric veins into the small portal branches of the liver, via the portal vein, in the pre-sinusoidal periportal tissues. In these sites, granulomas form around the eggs, leading to hepato-splenomegaly. Severe periportal fibrosis can follow the granuloma formation, with deposition of collagen around the portal vein and occlusion of the smaller portal branches. When this occurs, damage is usually irreversible [1].

In the case of *S. haematobium infestation*, worms stabilise in the pelvic venous plexus, and the symptoms and pathological changes of urogenital schistosomiasis are linked with oviposition in bladder tissue and genital organs. Oviposition is followed by intense inflammatory reactions and tissue eosinophilia, damage of the epithelial surface, ulceration and bleeding. The intense egg-induced tissue inflammation can result in bladder wall thickening and development of masses [1]. When inflammation and granuloma formation occur around the ostium of the ureter in the bladder blocking the passage of urine, hydronephrosis can occur, leading, in some cases, to renal insufficiency [1]. Finally, as a result of the inflammatory burden, Schistosome haematobium infestation can also have sequelae of oncological interest, and the parasite is among the ten infectious agents classified as carcinogens to human by IARC predisposing to Schistosoma-related bladder carcinomas [13].

Schistosome worms and egg oviposition in ectopic sites can cause site-specific manifestations and symptoms. In the case of neuro-schistosomiasis, encephalitis, epilepsy or transverse neuritis was described [1]. In the case of pulmonary schistosomiasis, the clinical features are caused by portal-cava shunting, transport of eggs to the lung capillaries and granuloma formation in the perialveolar area. The resulting fibrosis can cause pulmonary hypertension and cor-pulmonale due to increased pressure in the lung capillaries [1]. Another ectopic location of Schistosome infection consists of oviposition in female genital apparatus, occurring in approximately half of infected female. Tube-ovarian abscess, pelvic adhesions, ovarian cysts, ectopic pregnancy, tumour mimicking lesions or infertility was descried in these cases [12].

Cardiovascular involvement, which is the core topic of this book, can be considered among the ectopic sites of Schistosomiasis and will be analysed in detail in the dedicated paragraph of this chapter.

Diagnosis

Chronic schistosomiasis can be diagnosed by different methods. Direct methods rely on the visualization of parasite eggs by optical microscopy in different samples, including stool and urine, but also in semen, biopsies of bladder wall, liver, intestine and tissues of lower female genital tract [1, 7], when ectopic oviposition is suspected. According to the professional experience of the analyst, microscopy-based methods show a specificity of 100% while sensitivity varies with the intensity of infection, the concentration technique and number of samples examined and can be less than 50%, especially in patients with a low burden of infection [7]. A second type of direct diagnostic tool is represented by monoclonal antibody-based antigen detection techniques. These antigens, called circulating cathodic antigens, are produced in and released from the living worm intestine; as such, they are a sign of active infection, and their concentration is proportional to the worm burden. Antigen detection tools are suitable both for diagnosis and for follow-up of treatment response. Its sensitivity, compared to microscopy, varies according to the prevalence and intensity of infection and is higher for *S. mansoni* (72–89%) with respect to *S. haematobium* (24–39%) [7]. Circulating antigens can be detected before the worms have started producing eggs [1].

Schistosoma DNA in specimens potentially containing eggs or worms can be detected through real-time PCR, loop-mediated isothermal amplification and recombinase polymerase amplification, with a specificity reaching 100% and a sensitivity of 50%. This method can detect infection even in cases of negative microscopy [1, 7]. Serology is usually employed to determine whether or not a subject has been previously exposed to *Schistosoma* spp. infection. Seroconversion generally occurs within 4–8 weeks of infection up to 22 weeks. Sensitivity of sero-essays is higher if compared to optical microscopy assessment. Commercial kits can be based on different methods including immune-chromatography test, ELISA, Western Blot and indirect haemagglutination test [7].

Finally, ultrasonography can be used to visualize pathological changes associated with established active and late chronic schistosomiasis and the related organ-specific pathological changes, such as periportal fibrosis and signs of portal hypertension in intestinal schistosomiasis and bladder wall abnormalities and hydronephrosis in *S. haematobium* infection [1].

Prevention, Control and Treatment

According to the recently released WHO guidelines 2022 for prevention and control of schistosomiasis, in communities with a prevalence of *Schistosoma* spp. infection ≥10%, the annual preventive chemotherapy with a single dose of praziquantel at ≥75% treatment is recommended, with a coverage in all age groups from 2 years old, including adults, pregnant women after the first trimester and lactating women, to control schistosomiasis morbidity and work towards eliminating the disease as a public health problem. The frequency of distribution can be increased to biannual in case of non-response despite adequate coverage. WHO additionally recommends that health facilities provide access to treatment with praziquantel to control morbidity due to schistosomiasis in all infected individuals regardless of age, including pregnant women (excluding the first trimester), lactating women and children younger than 2 years (in this younger population, treatment should be based on testing and clinical judgement). Finally, in a perspective of integration approach towards control and elimination, WHO recommends water, sanitation and hygiene interventions, together with environmental interventions, including water engineering and focal snail control with molluscicides, and behavioural change interventions [14]. Praziquantel is the first-line antiparasitic treatment for schistosomiasis. Its dosage for chronic schistosomiasis is of 40 mg/kg/day orally in one or two divided doses the same day for *S. haematobium* e *S. mansoni* and 60 mg/kg/day in three divided doses the same day for *S. japonicum* e *S. mekongi* [7]. Data from south Saharan Africa report an average 75% cure rate and 85–95% egg reduction rate after a single intake of praziquantel [7].

Vascular Damage in Patients with Schistosomiasis

As introduced in previous paragraphs, the migration of *Schistosoma* spp. eggs outside the usual gastrointestinal and urinary excretion route, along with their entrapment in ectopic tissues, was documented in different anatomic regions [12], including the spleen, skin and central nervous system, [1], lungs in case of portal-cava shunting [1] and female genital apparatus, including tubes and ovaries [12]. Among the ectopic sites of oviposition, cardiovascular [8] and cerebrovascular involvement was described in previous cases and case series in literature [9], which were recently reviewed by our group.

Cardiovascular lesions were reported in cases in literature of patients with schistosomiasis, in the form of hemodynamic impairment (as portal or pulmonary hypertension), or arterial damage, such as aneurysm lesions [8, 15]. The results of our population-based exploratory study conducted among residents of Kome island, Tanzania, which consisted of the colour-Doppler ultrasound assessment of carotid and abdominal aorta of participants living in a region known to be endemic for schistosomiasis, provide useful inputs that could support both the haemodynamic pathophysiology perspective and the arterial damage perspective. Findings showed that a positive history of previous schistosomiasis infection was associated with an increase in maximum latero-lateral abdominal aorta diameter (aOR of 1.150 [95% CI: 1038–1274, $p = 0.007$]), suggesting that among populations endemic for schistosomiasis, non-atherosclerotic factors could contribute to cardiovascular damage. Additionally, an inverse association between diastolic blood pressure and history of previous schistosomiasis was observed, (aOR of 0.98 [95% CI: 0.95–0.99, $p = 0.04$]). As observed in patients with other pathological conditions known to impact cardiovascular risk, such as diabetes, the decrease in diastolic pressure could be caused by changes in elastic recoil, stiffness and compliance of the arteries [10].

In accordance with a recent systematic review and meta-analysis of the natural history of abdominal aortic ectasia, which shows no significant difference in terms of long-term risk between ectasia and aneurysm lesions [16], we consider the observed increase in aortic diameters among populations chronically exposed *Schistosoma* spp. as a call to reinforce prevention and control measurements for the parasitic infection, together with an integration of ongoing programs with cardiovascular prevention interventions and with a vascular morbidity management plan. Similarly, the inverse association found in logistic regression analysis between diastolic blood pressure and a previous history of schistosomiasis also supports the need for a strategy for cardiovascular prevention and control that could assess cardiological function, directly linked to vessel's integrity and physiology [10].

Pathophysiology of Vascular Lesions in Schistosomiasis

Several pathophysiological mechanisms were suggested to potentially underly vascular lesions in patients with schistosomiasis. The direct arterial wall damage due to obliterative endarteritis involving vasa vasorum or to contiguity with a focus of inflammation in surrounding tissues can occur [8, 17]. Additionally, a vasculitis process has been described in intra- and extracranial carotid arteries, potentially leading to stroke [9].

Granuloma formations are at the centre of the pathophysiological damage in districts that are reached by schistosome eggs. In the case of cardiovascular involvement, when chronic granulomatous inflammation caused by the embolized eggs affects the arteriolar districts, it can lead to haemodynamic impairment in the perfused organs. As an example, we can consider how the increased share stress secondary to the pulmonary hypertension can cause cardiac damage in the form of right ventricular dilatation and cor-pulmonale [17]. These haemodynamic changes can lead to structural damage of the involved vessels, including aneurysm formation. It was Zaky in 1962 who well described how hemodynamic changes occurring in patient with schistosomiasis could lead to aneurysm formation, by reporting a case series of pulmonary aneurysms occurring in patients affected by this parasitic condition [18]. According to his report, the repeated *Schistosoma* spp. oviposition causes a rise in arterial pressure and a consequent local weakening of the vessel wall; in this context, aneurysms are a late result of the haemodynamic conditions caused by the change in the arterial wall structure [18].

In addition to the haemodynamic mechanism described earlier, *Schistosoma* spp. eggs embolization may directly damage the walls of arteries by causing an obliterative endarteritis of their vasa vasorum, by damaging directly the endothelium or inducing atheromatic degeneration [19]. The direct damage to the endothelium and vessel wall by *Schistosome* eggs was well described by Vanker. Eggs of *Schistosoma mansoni* that spread from the left upper lobe of the lung to the adjacent pleura and to the aortic thoracic sheath can cause an endarteritis obliterans of those vasa vasorum that irrorate the thoracic aorta and, later on, favour the formation of an aneurysm in the weakened arterial wall [19]. Interestingly, this physio-pathological mechanism is shared by other infectious diseases associated with thoracic aortic aneurysms, such as tertiary syphilis [20].

Finally, a lesion can be caused through the direct damage due to contiguity with a focus on inflammation in surrounding tissues [17].

The same pathophysiological mechanisms described for the major vessel damage, such as lesions occurring in the aorta, can also explain the damage occurring to visceral arteries. In these cases, the haemodynamic impairment due to hepatic fibrosis and portal hypertension or as direct damage to the artery wall due to local inflammation can lead to visceral arteries aneurysms [21, 22].

Among all ectopic manifestations of schistosomiasis, a special consideration should be reserved to the vascular aspects of neuro-schistosomiasis. Cerebrovascular manifestations were described in the form of watershed infarction and cerebral vasculitis during primary *Schistosoma* infestation [23–25], or as a delayed manifestation of chronic infestation [26, 27]. Egg embolization in ectopic location, specifically in the nervous system, can lead, through inflammation, to neurological clinical manifestations [28, 29]; additionally, the suppressed immune responses towards viral and bacterial antigens can exacerbate the clinical presentation through the additional burden of overlapping infections [28].

Among the vascular changes that have been described in the literature in cerebral schistosomiasis caused by *S. mansoni* infestation, we can consider arteritis with fibrinoid necrosis involving the arterial wall, with or without ova or granulomatous lesions. Reports in literature related to specimens from cases of cerebrovascular schistosomiasis describe findings that include arterial wall thinning, interruption of the internal elastic membrane, aneurysmal dilatation, intimal thickening and vascular wall destruction with perivascular lympho-histiocytic infiltrate [30]. Cerebrovascular damage is not limited to the direct effect of infection, but can also be iatrogenic. It was reported that praziquantel treatment can occasionally affect the cerebrovascular status in treated patients, through the *Schistosoma* lysis induced by the drug, which triggers an immunological reaction [25].

The case that best describes cerebrovascular pathology in schistosomiasis was published by Camuset et al., which described both the carotid artery involvement in schistosomiasis and the iatrogenic effects of praziquantel treatment on cerebrovascular districts. The report contains the history of a 28-year-old female patient returning from Burkina Faso with hemiplegia and language disorders, a junctional infarction, carotid stenosis and a contralateral carotid inflammation. After a second course of praziquantel, a new stenosis of the right carotid siphon was diagnosed on magnetic resonance imaging, secondary to the exacerbation of carotid vasculitis. The resolution of the clinical picture, in this case, was acquired with intra-venous methylprednisolone therapy [26].

Even though the vascular involvement in the form of cerebral [30] or carotid artery vasculitis with stenosis [26] was described in patients with schistosomiasis symptomatic for stroke [26, 27], up until now no lesions requiring a surgical management were described in literature [9].

A pictorial view of the pathophysiology mechanisms behind the formation of pulmonary and aortic aneurysms and visceral aneurysms is available in Figs. 2.1 and 2.2, respectively (pathophysiological mechanisms behind vascular lesions in patients with schistosomiasis were described).

Clinical Presentation

The clinical cases of aneurysms occurring in patients with schistosomiasis and published in literature were recently revised by our group. A summary of the clinical presentation of the revised cases, reproduced from the previous publication, is available in Table 2.1. According to the review findings, it was observed that the age at diagnosis is younger if compared to patients with atherosclerotic aneurysms and frequently younger than 40 years [18, 19, 31–33]. This fact suggests the need for an increased clinical suspicion for aneurysm as differential diagnosis when assessing patients of young age presenting with a compatible clinical presentation in endemic areas [8].

The most frequently reported symptom in reviewed reports of patients with aneurysm and a history of schistosomiasis was pain, which could be referred to the chest, to the hypochondrium or to the lumbar region, followed by dyspnoea, fever, hoarseness and Ortner's syndrome, hyper-eosinophilia, syncope, cardiogenic shock

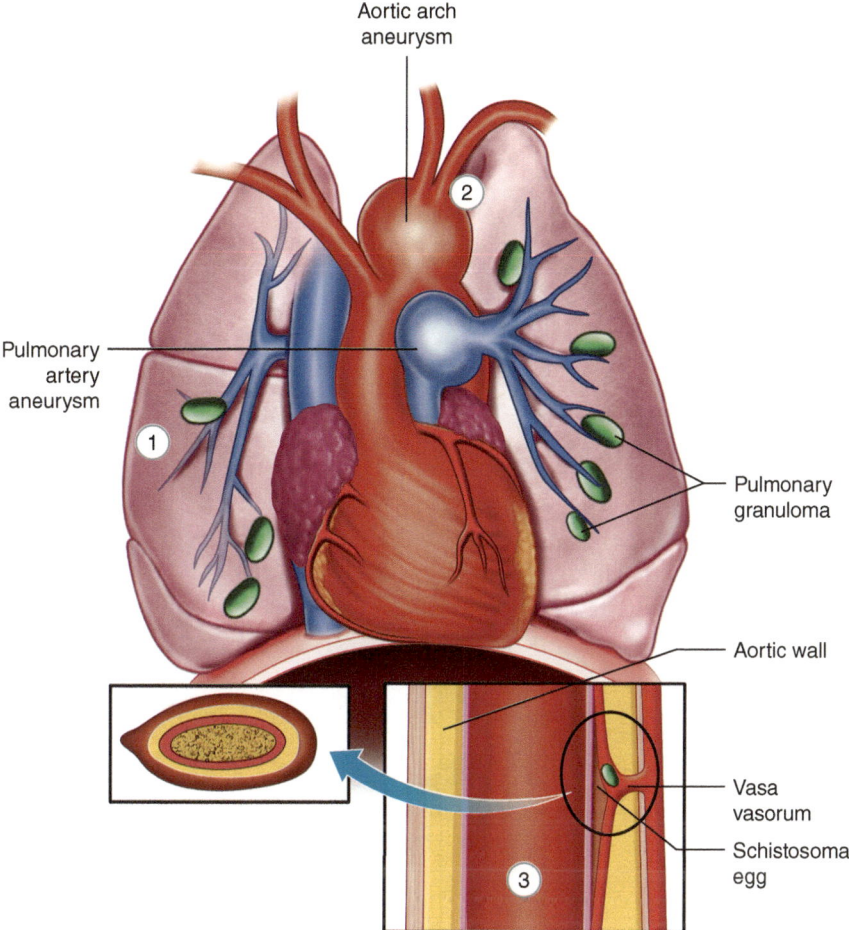

Fig. 2.1 Aneurysms and Schistosomiasis. Physiopathology behind aortic aneurysm and pulmonary artery aneurysm formation. (1) Schistosoma eggs may seed pulmonary arteries, leading to lung inflammatory reaction, granuloma formation. Direct damage to vessels may occur as a result of inflammation of tissues surrounding vessels. (2) Pulmonary inflammation due to Schistosoma eggs seeding of pulmonary arteries may lead to pulmonary hypertension. Damage to vessels may be due to hemodynamic changes. (3) Schistosoma eggs may seed major vessels wall through vasa vasorum, causing cystic medial necrosis and loss of wall integrity. The figure is original work by the author VS, previously published in . Silvestri V, Mushi V, Mshana MI, Bonaventura WM, Justine NC, Sabas D, et al. Blood Flukes and Arterial Damage: A Review of Aneurysm Cases in Patients with Schistosomiasis. Vol. 2022, Canadian Journal of Infectious Diseases and Medical Microbiology. 2022 [8]

and anaemia [8]. Cardiovascular issues were the most frequent associated preexistent co-morbidities, including hypertension, previous surgery for aortic pathology (type A aortic dissection in one case), oesophageal varices and a history of smoke and alcohol consumption [8].

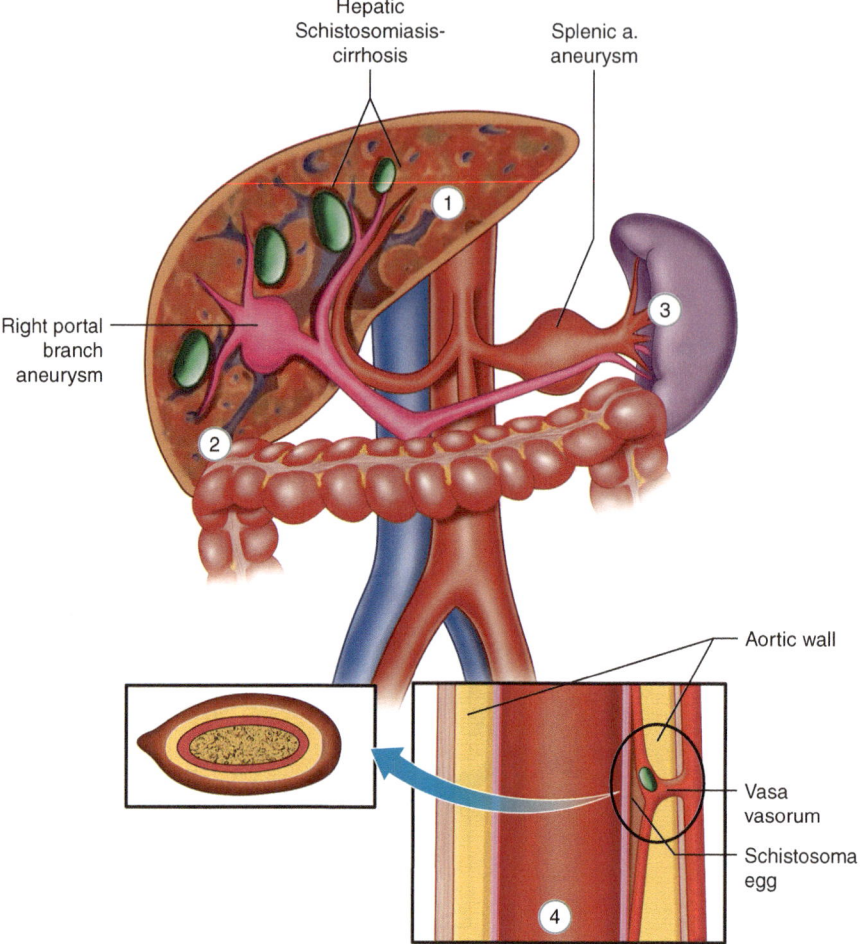

Fig. 2.2 Aneurysms and Schistosomiasis. Physiopathology behind portal branch aneurysm and splenic artery aneurysm formation. (1) Seeding of hepatic vessels by Schistosoma eggs may lead to inflammatory reaction in hepatic parenchyma, fibrosis and direct damage to vessels. (2) Inflammatory reaction and portal fibrosis due to Schistosoma oviposition in hepatic vessels may lead to portal hypertension, which may induce aneurysms by hemodynamic mechanisms in visceral vessels. (3) Splenic artery aneurysm may be secondary to portal hypertension. (4) Schistosoma eggs may seed arterial wall through vasa vasorum, inducing direct damage and predisposing to aneurysm formation. *Splenic a.* splenic artery. Figures 2 and 3 are adapted from the original art work by the author V.S, previously published in Silvestri V, Mushi V, Mshana MI, Bonaventura WM, Justine NC, Sabas D, et al. Blood Flukes and Arterial Damage: A Review of Aneurysm Cases in Patients with Schistosomiasis. Vol. 2022, Canadian Journal of Infectious Diseases and Medical Microbiology. 2022 [8]

Table 2.1 Summary of cases

N	Author, year	Age, sex	Geographic region	Schistosoma species	Comorbidities and c.v. risk factors in Anamnesis	Schistosomiasis details	Clinical presentation	Vascular findings	Pharmacological treatment of schistosomiasis
1	Salah, 1997	27, M	Egypt	n.a.	Smoke	Previous urinary and intestinal schistosomiasis Normal lung parenchima	Cardio-vocal Ortner's syndrome; exertional dyspnoea (2 months) Pulmonary hypertension	Pulmonary artery- aneurysm And schistosomal Cor pulmonale	Previous treatment with praziquantel for intestinal and urinary schistosomiasis
2	Vanker, 1986	19, F	South-Africa	*Schistosoma mansoni* (stool and rectal mucosa)	None	Pulmonary shistosomiasis	Haemoptysis; left chest pain, hoarseness, absent left brachial pulse (1 month) Haematuria	Aortic arch pseudoaneurysm (7 × 2 cm)	Not reported
3	Mucenic, 2002	45, M	Lived for 17 years in *Schistosoma* endemic area	Negative (stool and rectal biopsy)	No other	Previous hepatosplenic schistosomiasis (hematemesis, enterorrhagia, oesophageal varices)	Abdominal continuous pain (left hypochondrium)	Right portal branch aneurysm (5 × 4 × 4 cm)	No previous treatment with praziquantel

(continued)

Table 2.1 (continued)

N	Author, year	Age, sex	Geographic region	Schistosoma species	Comorbidities and c.v. risk factors in Anamnesis	Schistosomiasis details	Clinical presentation	Vascular findings	Pharmacological treatment of schistosomiasis
4	Lambertucci, 2010	66, F	Brazil	n.a.	No other	Chronic Hepato-splenic schistosomiasis (Esophago-gastric varices; hematemesis)	Routine assessment for hepato-splenic schistosomiasis	Saccular aneurysm of the splenic artery; intra-hepatic shunt between right portal branch-and right hepatic vein	Beta-blockers as gastroenteric haemorrhage prophylaxis
5	Piveta, 2012	41, F	Brazil	n.a.	Alcoholic hepatitis Waiting for liver transplant	Hepato-splenic schistosomiasis	Intermittent chest pain; Pulmonary hypertension; intra-pulmonary shunt	Pulmonary a. aneurysm (8.3 cm)	Not reported
6	Genzini, 2014	48, M	Brazil	n.a.	Hypertension, thrombo-cytopenia	Advanced hepatosplenic schistosomiasis	Right lumbar pain	Right renal artery aneurysm 2.5 cm	Not reported
7	Ramadan, 2015	55, M	Lower-Egypt	*Schistosoma mansoni* (lung biopsy)	Ex-smoker	History of intestinal and hepato-splenic schistosomiasis. Pulmonary granuloma Positive serology S. mansoni	Dyspnoea (one month); fever (2 months) cough and mucoid sputum (10 days) left atrial compression; Pleural effusion	Right pulmonary artery aneurysm (17 × 11 cm)	Previous treatment for intestinal schistosomiasis (20 years previously). Anti-coagulation

8	Abdelnaby, 2018	50, F	Egypt	n.a.	n.a.	Bilharziasis since early childhood	Chest pain (recurrent); exertional dyspnoea	Right and left pulmonary a. aneurysm (6.5 cm) and atrial mural thrombus	Anticoagulation
9	Athanazio, 2018	n.a., M	Brazil	*Schistosoma mansoni* (lung, testis, liver, large bowl)	n.a.	Testicular, intestinal and lung schistosomiasis	Spontaneous aorto-cutaneous fistula	Thoraco-abdominal aortic aneurysm; spontaneous aorto-cutaneous fistula	n.a.
10	Gavilanes, 2018	38, M	Brazil	n.a.	n.a.	Chronic schistosomiasis, pulmonary artery hypertension	Palpitations; dyspnoea; exertional syncope	Giant pulmonary artery aneurysm; Aorta and left coronary artery compression	n.a.
11	De Oliveira, 2019	48, M	Brazil	n.a.	Type A aortic dissection ascending aorta substitution (Dacron); biological valve	Hepato-splenic schistosomiasis	Fever *Porphyromonas pogonae* sepsis	Aortic graft infection and aortic rupture	Antibiotics for associated bacteria

(continued)

Table 2.1 (continued)

N	Author, year	Age, sex	Geographic region	Schistosoma species	Comorbidities and c.v. risk factors in Anamnesis	Schistosomiasis details	Clinical presentation	Vascular findings	Pharmacological treatment of schistosomiasis
12	Dyer, 2020	18, F	Australia	*Schistosoma* Ag EIA	n.a	Serology positive for Schistosomiasis	Fever; right upper quadrant pain; liver abscess *Fasciola hepatica* infestation	Hepatic artery pseudoaneurysm; acute bleeding from the ampulla of Vater	Praziquantel
13	Abdelnaby, 2020	38, F	Egypt	n.a.		History of bilharzias	Dyspnoea (5 years) and hoarseness (1 year)	Pulmonary artery aneurysm (PAA) with dilatation of both branches and hoarseness	Anticoagulation

Anagraphic details, geographic region of patient's origin/residency, schistosomiasis details, clinical presentation, vascular findings and pharmacological management

M male, *F* female, *Ag EIA* antigen enzyme-linked immunosorbent essay, *n.a.* not available, *C.v.* cardio-vascular

The most frequently involved arterial district was the pulmonary artery, followed by aortic lesions which included one recurrent lesion on previous aortic surgery and abdominal visceral vessels aneurysms (specifically in splenic, hepatic artery, right portal branch and renal artery). Available at Silvestri V, Mushi V, Mshana MI, Bonaventura WM, Justine NC, Sabas D, et al. Blood Flukes and Arterial Damage: A Review of Aneurysm Cases in Patients with Schistosomiasis. Vol. 2022, Canadian Journal of Infectious Diseases and Medical Microbiology. 2022 [8]

A history of previously diagnosed schistosomiasis or a chronic schistosomiasis was reported in the majority of cases, but occasionally aneurysms occurred in patients who had lived in endemic areas previously to the vascular diagnosis and many years after leaving the endemic country [8].

The most frequently involved arterial district was the pulmonary artery, followed by aortic lesions which included one recurrent lesions on previous aortic surgery and cases of abdominal visceral vessels aneurysms (specifically in splenic, hepatic artery, right portal branch and renal artery) [8].

Among the complications of arterial lesions, thrombophilia was reported in some cases. Abdelnaby described a pulmonary artery aneurysm that was complicated by atrial mural thrombus [15], and Ramadan reported on a massive pulmonary embolism which complicated a pulmonary artery aneurysm [17]. Mucenic described the post-operatory for splenectomy in a patient with hepatic artery aneurysm as complicated by partial spleen vein thrombosis. The inflammation-induced thrombophilia that is associated with schistosomiasis could be the factor favouring the formation of thrombus in the aneurysm lumen, suggesting that secondary thrombophilia should thus be considered an additional cardiovascular risk factor in the clinical context of aneurysms occurring in patients affected by this parasitic disease [8].

The histological findings from the published cases supported the pathophysiological mechanisms suggested by several authors to explain the co-occurrence of arterial lesions in this parasitic disease, as analysed in the previous chapter. Histological findings showed that *Schistosome* granuloma formations can occur in both the arterial wall and surrounding organs. It is the case of the aortic wall affected by aortic arch pseudoaneurysm, in which *Schistosoma* eggs surrounded by a granulomatous reaction were found on histological examination in the pulmonary parenchyma, in the pleura and in arterioles [19]. Similarly, in the case of a thoraco-abdominal aortic aneurysm, the histology revealed eggs in the liver, large bowl and calcified eggs in the lung and testis [34].

Eggs were not always detected in specimens, as in a case of a right portal branch aneurysm, splenic and liver fibrosis, in which the destruction of portal vein branches was observed, even though *Schistosoma* eggs could not be found in the samples [22].

Surgical Management and Outcome

Different kinds of surgical approaches were described according to the location of the aneurysm [8]. A summary of the surgical approaches used in the cases in literature, previously published in a review from our group [8], is available in Table 2.2.

Aneurysmectomy and direct suture were used to treat an aortic arch pseudoaneurysm by Vanker [34]. Nefrectomy, aneurysmectomy and renal reimplantation were described as successful in a renal artery aneurysm [35]. Splenectomy was considered in a portal branch aneurysm associated with portal hypertension. In this last case, by reducing portal hypertension, splenectomy favoured the reduction of aneurysm size to 1.4 cm at 4-year follow-up [22], suggesting that the excessive venous inflow from the splenic vein could contribute to portal hypertension and vessel

Table 2.2 *Surgical* treatment and outcome of patients

N	Author, year	Age, sex	Vascular findings	Surgical treatment	Outcome
2	Vanker, 1986	19, F	Aortic arch pseudoaneurysm (7 × 2 cm)	Aneurysmectomy and direct suture	Unknown
3	Mucenic, 2002	45, M	Right portal branch aneurysm (5 × 4 × 4 cm)	Splenectomy	Partial portal vein thrombosis Alive (reduction of aneurysm size to 1.4 cm and resolution of the vessel thrombosis on follow up)
4	Lambertucci, 2010	66, F	Saccular aneurysm of the splenic artery; intra-hepatic shunt between right portal branch-and right hepatic vein	Refused surgery Treated with beta-blockers	Unknown
5	Piveta, 2012	41, F	Pulmonary artery aneurysm (8.3 cm)	Exitus waiting for surgery	Exitus (Aneurysm rupture and cardiac tamponade)
6	Genzini, 2014	48, M	Right renal artery aneurysm (2.5 cm)	Nephrectomy, aneurysmectomy and renal reimplantation	Alive (creatinine improvement on follow-up)
7	Ramadan, 2015	55, M	Right pulmonary artery aneurysm (17 × 11 cm)	Refused surgery On anti-coagulation	Exitus (massive pulmonary embolization, notwithstanding anti-coagulant therapy)
11	De Oliveira 2019	48 M	Aortic graft infection and aortic rupture	Not-specified reintervention on previous aortic graft On antibiotic therapy	Exitus (complications of surgery on 12th day post-operatory, likely due to comorbidities related to hepato-splenic schistosomiasis)
12	Dyer 2020	18, F	Hepatic artery pseudoaneurysm; acute bleeding from the ampulla of Vater	Not specified In therapy with praziquantel and	Bleeding of aneurysm from Vater ampulla, notwithstanding praziquantel
13	Abdelnaby, 2020	38, F	Pulmonary artery aneurysm with dilatation of both branches and Ortner's syndrome	Refused surgery	Discharged on close follow-up

Anagraphical details, aneurysm description, surgical management and outcome of patients were specified. Fatality was reported in 3/13 patients

F female, *M* male

Available at Silvestri V, Mushi V, Mshana MI, Bonaventura WM, Justine NC, Sabas D, et al. Blood Flukes and Arterial Damage: A Review of Aneurysm Cases in Patients with Schistosomiasis. Vol. 2022, Canadian Journal of Infectious Diseases and Medical Microbiology. 2022 [8]

dilatation [22], and aneurysm lesions may be prone to reduction in size when the haemodynamic condition that favours their development is treated. One option to achieve this goal is the implant of a trans-jugular intrahepatic portosystemic shunt, a reversible and less invasive alternative to surgery in patients with portal hypertension, including the one due to *Schistosoma* infection (Fig. 2.3). This percutaneous technique can preserve the spleen and its immunologic function [36]. The limited availability in an endemic setting, the high cost and the marginal indications in guidelines were suggested as factors that challenge the assessment of the safety and effectiveness of this technique in the low-resource settings which are endemic for NTDs [8, 37].

When it comes to giving an indication for surgery, some specific features of aneurysms in patients with schistosomiasis should be considered. The local weakening of the aneurysm wall due to the ongoing haemodynamic changes, as in the case of the rise of pressure, and to the implantation of *Schistosoma* ova in tissue was exhaustively described previously [38]. This impairment in the physiological structure of the aortic wall and its weakened structure can increase the risk of arterial (and aneurysm) rupture [39]. It should be emphasized that rupture can complicate an aneurysm lesion in patients with schistosomiasis, notwithstanding the treatment of the underlying parasitic condition with the anti-parasitic praziquantel [32].

In addition to the quality of the vessels wall, to the increased risk of rupture, the surgical indication and planning should also consider the risk of thrombophilia-related complications, as described in the previous section [8]. Another challenge for surgery is linked to the patient's general conditions, which are frequently

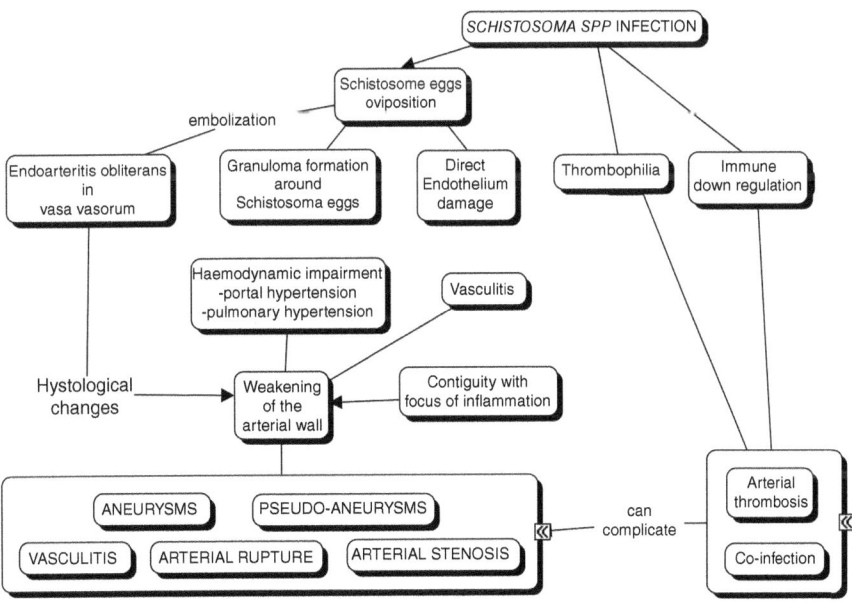

Fig. 2.3 Schistosoma spp. infection: pathophysiology of vascular damage

impaired by additional cardiovascular dysfunction in the form of pulmonary or portal hypertension. The effects of *Schistosoma*-induced immune-modulation [40], which can increase the risk for overlapping infections [39] or sepsis [40], are another concern for surgical management. Finally, we shouldn't forget that the clinical features can be exacerbated by malnutrition, which can be significantly prevalent in endemic areas [38].

Conclusions and Recommendations

Features of aortic structural damage and haemodynamic impairment, along with arterial aneurysm lesions were described in patients with a history of schistosomiasis or in cases affected by an ongoing *Schistosome* spp. infection. Findings are a call to integrate programmes with a cardiovascular prevention and a morbidity management plan. Additional factors linked to cardiovascular morbidity, as the parasite-induced immune downregulation and the consequent increased co-infection risk or the *Schistosome*-induced thrombophilia, should be considered when planning surgical treatment in these patients and promptly managed to reduce their impact on the patient's outcome. Further studies are needed to fully understand the features of vascular interest in schistosomiasis, to better inform the clinical and surgical management in endemic settings.

Acknowledgements This chapter was based on two previous reviews and one original research published by our group: Silvestri V, Mushi V, Mshana MI, Bonaventura WM, Justine NC, Sabas D, Ngasala B. Blood Flukes and Arterial Damage: A Review of Aneurysm Cases in Patients with Schistosomiasis. Can J Infect Dis Med Microbiol. 2022 Dec 3;2022:6483819; Silvestri V, Mushi V, Ngasala B, Kihwele J, Sabas D, Rocchi L. Stroke in Patients with Schistosomiasis: Review of Cases in Literature. Can J Infect Dis Med Microbiol. 2022 Jul 25;2022:3902570; Silvestri V, Mshana MI, Mushi V, Bonaventura WM, Justine NC, Kinabo C, Zacharia A, La Torre G, Ngasala B. Subclinical vascular damage in Schistosoma spp. endemic regions. Vasa. 2023 Mar 22.

References

1. McManus DP, Dunne DW, Sacko M, Utzinger J, Vennervald BJ, Zhou X-NN. Schistosomiasis. Nat Rev Dis Prim. 2018;4(1):1–19.
2. Mawa PA, Kincaid-Smith J, Tukahebwa EM, Webster JP, Wilson S. Schistosomiasis morbidity hotspots: roles of the human host, the parasite and their Interface in the development of severe morbidity. Front Immunol. 2021;12(12):635869.
3. Ziskind B. La bilharziose urinaire en ancienne Égypte. Nephrol Ther. 2009;5(7):658–61.
4. Di Bella S, Riccardi N, Giacobbe DR. History of schistosomiasis (bilharziasis) in humans: from Egyptian medical papyri to molecular biology on mummies. Pathog Glob Health. 2018;112(5):268–73. https://doi.org/10.1080/20477724.2018.1495357.
5. Yeh HY, Zhan X, Qi W. A comparison of ancient parasites as seen from archeological contexts and early medical texts in China. Int J Paleopathol. 2019;25:30–8. https://doi.org/10.1016/j.ijpp.2019.03.004.
6. Mazigo HD, Nuwaha F, Kinung'Hi SM, Morona D, De Moira AP, Wilson S, et al. Epidemiology and control of human schistosomiasis in Tanzania. Parasites Vectors. 2012;5(1):1.

7. Comelli A, Genovese C, Gobbi F, Brindicci G, Capone S, Corpolongo A, et al. Schistosomiasis in non-endemic areas: Italian consensus recommendations for screening, diagnosis and management by the Italian Society of Tropical Medicine and Global Health (SIMET), endorsed by the Committee for the Study of Parasitology of the Italian A. Infection. 2023;51(5):1249–71. https://doi.org/10.1007/s15010-023-02050-7.

8. Silvestri V, Mushi V, Mshana MI, Bonaventura WM, Justine NC, Sabas D, et al. Blood flukes and arterial damage: a review of aneurysm cases in patients with schistosomiasis. Can J Infect Dis Med Microbiol. 2022;2022:2022.

9. Silvestri V, Mushi V, Ngasala B, Kihwele J, Sabas D, Rocchi L. Stroke in patients with schistosomiasis: review of cases in literature. Can J Infect Dis Med Microbiol. 2022;2022:3902570.

10. Silvestri V, Mshana MI, Mushi V, Bonaventura WM, Justine NC, Kinabo C, et al. Subclinical vascular damage in Schistosoma spp. endemic regions: a community based cross-sectional study in Kome Island, Tanzania. Vasa Eur J Vasc Med. 2023:1–9.

11. Lo NC, Bezerra FSM, Colley DG, Fleming FM, Homeida M, Kabatereine N, et al. Review of 2022 WHO guidelines on the control and elimination of schistosomiasis. Lancet Infect Dis. 2022;22(11):e327–35.

12. Elias E, Silvestri V, Mushi V, Mandarano M. Ovarian schistosomiasis: challenges of a neglected ectopic involvement of blood flukes. Case report and review of literature. Pathologica. 2023;115(4):237–45.

13. Salim EI, Morimura K, Menesi A, El-lity M. Elevated oxidative stress and DNA damage and repair levels in urinary bladder carcinomas associated with Schistosomiasis. Int J Cancer. 2008;608:601–8.

14. Wiegand RE, Fleming FM, de Vlas SJ, Odiere MR, Kinung'hi S, King CH, et al. Defining elimination as a public health problem for schistosomiasis control programmes: beyond prevalence of heavy-intensity infections. Lancet Glob Heal. 2022;10(9):e1355–9.

15. Abdelnaby M, Almaghraby A, Saleh Y, Ziada K. A bilharzial pulmonary artery aneurysm with a large calcified mural thrombus. Int J Cardiovasc Imaging. 2019;35(3):549–50.

16. Shirasu T, Takagi H, Kuno T, Yasuhara J, Kent KC, Tracci MC, et al. Risk of rupture and all-cause mortality of abdominal aortic ectasia: a systematic review and meta-analysis. Eur J Vasc Endovasc Surg. 2022;177(2):566–8.

17. Abo-Salem ES, Ramadan MM. A huge thrombosed pulmonary artery aneurysm without pulmonary hypertension in a patient with hepatosplenic schistosomiasis. Am J Case Rep. 2015;16:140–5.

18. Gavilanes F, Piloto B, Fernandes CJC. Giant pulmonary artery aneurysm in a patient with schistosomiasis-associated pulmonary arterial hypertension. J Bras Pneumol. 2018;44(2):167.

19. Vanker EA. Aortic aneurysm caused by schistosomiasis. Thorax. 1986;41(11):890–1.

20. De Rango P, De Socio GV, Silvestri V, Simonte G, Verzini F. An unusual case of epigastric and back pain expanding descending thoracic aneurysm resulting from tertiary syphilis diagnosed with positron emission tomography. Circ Cardiovasc Imaging. 2013;6:1120–1.

21. Lambertucci JR, Voieta I, Andrade LM. Intrahepatic venous shunt and splenic artery aneurysm in hepatosplenic schistosomiasis. Rev Soc Bras Med Trop. 2010;43(2):215.

22. Mucenic M, de Souza RM, Atílio Laudanna A, Rocha Md Mde S, Laudanna AA, Cancado EL. Treatment by splenectomy of a portal vein aneurysm in hepatosplenic schistosomiasis. Rev Inst Med Trop Sao Paulo. 2002;44(5):261–4.

23. Sarazin M, Caumes E, Cohen A, Amarenco P. Multiple microembolic borderzone brain infarctions and endomyocardial fibrosis in idiopathic hypereosinophilic syndrome and in Schistosoma mansoni infestation. J Neurol Neurosurg Psychiatry. 2004;75(2):305–7.

24. Jauréguiberry S, Ansart S, Perez L, Danis M, Bricaire F, Caumes E. Acute neuroschistosomiasis: two cases associated with cerebral vasculitis. Am J Trop Med Hyg. 2007;76(5):964–6.

25. Grandière-Pérez L, Caumes E. Corticosteroids for watershed infarction in acute schistosomiasis. Clin Infect Dis. 2013;57(6):918–9.

26. Camuset G, Wolff V, Marescaux C, Abou-Bacar A, Candolfi E, Lefebvre N, et al. Cerebral vasculitis associated with Schistosoma mansoni infection. BMC Infect Dis. 2012;12:2–5.

27. Nyein AM, Sann AA, Aye NN, Tan CT. Delayed onset cerebral vasculitis from chronic schisto-
    soma mansoni infection in Myanmar: a case report. Neurol Asia. 2020;25(2):203–6.
28. Costain AH, Macdonald AS, Smits HH. Schistosome egg migration: mechanisms.
    Pathogenesis Host Immune Responses. 2018;9(December):1–16.
29. Nation CS, Da AA, Id JKM, Id PJS. Schistosome migration in the definitive host. PLoS Negl
    Trop Dis. 2020;14(4):4–6.
30. Berkowitz AL, Raibagkar P, Pritt BS, Mateen FJ. Neurologic manifestations of the
    neglected tropical diseases. J Neurol Sci. 2015;349(1–2):20–32. https://doi.org/10.1016/j.
    jns.2015.01.001.
31. Soliman MSEDS. Hoarseness in schistosomat cor pulmonale. Chest. 1997;112(4):1150.
32. Dyer J, Henderson A. A diagnostic fluke. Pathology. 2020;52:S50.
33. Abdelnabi M, Eshak N, Attia I, Abdelkader M, Saleh Y, Almaghraby A. Ortner's syndrome
    due to large bilharzial pulmonary artery aneurysm. Echocardiography. 2020;37(7):1109–10.
34. Athanazio DA, Athanazio PRF. Asymetric testicular schistosomal infection. Brazilian J Infect
    Dis. 2008;12(6):461.
35. Genzini T, Noujaim HM, Mota LT, Ianhez LE, de Oliveira RA, Shiroma ETM, et al.
    Autotransplante renal para tratamento de aneurisma de artéria renal: Relato de caso. Sao Paulo
    Med J. 2014;132(5):307–10.
36. Richter J, Bode JG, Blondin D, Kircheis G, Kubitz R, Holtfreter MC, et al. Severe liver fibrosis
    caused by Schistosoma mansoni: management and treatment with a transjugular intrahepatic
    portosystemic shunt. Lancet Infect Dis. 2015;15(6):731–7.
37. Kraef C, Arand J, Galaski J, Jordan S, Kluwe J, Lohse AW, et al. Transjugular Intrahepatic
    Portosystemic Shunt (TIPS) for primary and secondary prophylaxis of variceal bleeding in
    hepatic schistosomiasis. Travel Med Infect Dis. 2019;30:130–2.
38. Zaky HA. Aneurysm of the pulmonary artery due to schistosomiasis. Dis Chest.
    1952;21(2):194–204.
39. Piveta RB, Arruda AL, Rodrigues AC, Pinheiro JA, Andrade JL. Rupture of a giant aneurysm
    of the pulmonary artery caused by schistosomiasis. Eur Heart J. 2012;33(9):1159.
40. Romero de Oliveira A, Nürmberger JM, Issa M, Pinto V, MMK B, Rabelato JT, et al. Late
    ascending aortic prosthesis infection by Porphyromonas pogonae: an unexpected infectious
    complication. Anaerobe. 2019;56:106–8.

Hydatidosis

3

Contents

Introduction

Echinococcosis is a zoonotic helminthic disease caused by the metacestodes stage of *Echinococcus granulosus*, *E. multilocularis*, *E. vogeli* and *E. oligarthrus* [1]. It is included among the 20 neglected tropical diseases of global health importance recognized by WHO [2], The disease can have different clinical manifestations according to the species of Echinococcus involved; this disease group includes cystic, alveolar and neotropical echinococcosis. The etiologic agent of cystic echinococcosis is *Echinococcus granulosus* sensu lato, which has a worldwide distribution. *Echinococcus multilocularis,* which is the cause of alveolar echinococcosis, is endemic in the northern hemisphere. Finally, *Echinococcus vogeli* and *Echinococcus oligarthra,* which are responsible for neotropical echinococcosis, are restricted to Mexico, Central America and South America [3].

Hydatidosis in History

Echinococcosis is known to affect humans since antiquity. Due to the fact that hydatid cysts frequently undergo calcification, paleo-pathological studies were able to report on about 25 cases from 18 different sites, from the Hellenistic to the Post-Medieval periods, from both southern and northern Europe [4]. It is the case of the remains of an adolescent from the late Roman period buried in Amiens (Northern France) [5] or of the report of the cystic lesion found in the thoraco-abdominal region of a thirteenth-century adult female from the medieval cemetery of the Abbey of Pozzeveri (Lucca, Italy) [4]. The presence of hydatid cysts in the archaeological contexts can be connected with agro-pastoral practices and poor hygiene [4].

According to historical documents, we know that Hippocrates described hydatid cysts in the late fifth century BC, and that in the Middles Ages, during the tenth century, cystic echinococcosis was known to the Arabian physician Al-Rhazes [4]. Still it was only in the seventeenth century, precisely in 1684, that the Italian physician Francesco Redi recognized that the disease was caused by a parasitic infection [4]. This discovery followed the autopsy done by Redi on the body of the grand duke of Tuscany Ferdinando II de Medici, which showed that "*the lungs, bad in colour and consistency, were externally full of watery vesicles, which are called "hydatids" by the doctors [...]. At the base of the heart, there were many vesicles of different sizes full of water gathered together like a bunch of grapes*" [6].

With time, additional observations allowed a better understanding of the disease. In 1863, *E. multilocularis* was identified by Leuckart, and only during the early to mid-1900s, the more distinct features of its life cycle and how it cause disease were fully described and studied [4, 6].

Epidemiology

Cystic echinococcosis, caused by *Echinococcus granulosus* sensu lato, is a cosmopolitan disease, with an annual incidence ranging from 1 to 200 per 100,000 in endemic areas. Its mortality rate is approximately 2–4%, in cases where appropriate treatment is provided [7]. Dogs and other carnivores are the primary parasite's hosts, sheep are the intermediate ones, whereas humans can be accidental hosts of the parasite. Human infestation occurs by ingesting food, milk or water contaminated by dog faeces containing the ova of the parasite [8].

A recent systematic review by Casulli et al. identified approximately 65,000 human cystic echinococcosis cases in Europe during the past 25 years, with a mean annual incidence of 0·64 cases per 100,000 people, and emphasized that cystic echinococcosis remains a relevant public health issue in the Mediterranean Europe, specifically in Italy and Spain and in eastern and south-eastern European countries, with the Balkan Peninsula as the current focus of cystic echinococcosis in Europe [3]. In Africa, *E. granulosus* is widespread in domestic livestock including sheep, cattle and goats. Over 18 species of wild herbivores from different parts of southern, central and eastern Africa are infected with hydatid cysts [9]. Echinococcosis is endemic in sub-Saharan countries, with a higher prevalence reported than in other endemic settings. Serologic studies conducted in rural areas in Tanzania have reported a prevalence up to 11.5% [1].

Alveolar echinococcosis, caused by *Echinococcus multilocularis,* has a lower annual incidence, if compared to cystic echinococcosis, ranging from 0.03 to 1.2 per 100,000 but a higher mortality, which can reach 90% within 10–15 years of diagnosis [7]. It was estimated that for every human alveolar echinococcosis infection, 10–20 cystic echinococcosis infections can be expected, particularly in Europe but also worldwide [3]. Differently from cystic echinococcosis, which broadly affects Mediterranean Europe, alveolar echinococcosis is mainly prevalent in Asia. Casulli et al. reported that of the approximately 18,000 new cases per year of alveolar echinococcosis estimated globally, 91% of cases occur in China and around 1600 cases in Europe, central Asia and Russia [3].

Echinococcus multilocularis "evolved" with a successful wild, sylvatic life cycle involving foxes as definitive hosts and rodents as intermediate host. Initially endemic in the ecosystems of the Arctic tundra or Tibetan high-altitude grasslands, its life cycle is actually perfectly suited to transmission in an urban environment, through the increase in the number of foxes and rodents in urban areas and through spill-over to domestic hosts, making the urbanization of *E. multilocularis* a significant public health issue, particularly in Europe [9], but also Japan and more recently, in Canada, where both foxes and coyotes are involved in transmission of the parasite. In this context, the need to re-assess the role of dogs as an at risk definitive host in the epidemiology of *E. multilocularis* infections is actual and urgent [9].

Pathophysiology

In both cystic echinococcosis and alveolar echinococcosis, humans act as dead-end hosts through a hand-to-mouth and food-borne or water-borne transmission of infective eggs of the parasite [3]. The ingested ova release larvae, or onco-spheres, in the small intestine. After ingestion, cysts migrate through the portal venous system or through the lymphatic system, where they frequently get trapped into the hepatic sinusoids. Larvae that succeed in passing through the liver parenchyma reach the lungs and systemic circulation. Because of this route for dissemination, the liver and lungs are the sites most frequently involved by cystic lesions [10]. Cystic echinococcosis mainly affects these two organs, even though the parasite's cysts can involve any organ or tissue. The infestation is characterized by the occurrence of fluid-filled, isolated, parasitic cysts growing concentrically, and it can be asymptomatic or pauci-symptomatic for years. The absence of signs of acute infection might contribute to the underdiagnosis or to the delay in diagnosis of cases. The progressive growth of Echinococcus cysts might cause compression of neighbouring structures, which can lead to non-specific symptoms. In severe cases, the clinical scenario can be determined by symptoms and signs due to overlapping complications on the cystic lesions, such as rupture or superinfections. Such non-specific presentation of the disease challenges its prompt diagnosis and frequently, can lead to misdiagnosis [3].

Different are the clinical features of *Echinococcus multilocularis* infestation. This species is the aetiological agent of alveolar echinococcosis. The parasite's invasion is characterized by a metastasizing nature, making the disease one of the most potentially fatal zoonotic diseases in the Northern Hemisphere [9].

Diagnosis

Differently from other parasitic infections, the protective isolation of the parasite from the exposure to the immune system, which is possible inside its cystic structures, can impair the triggering of a detectable antibody response, which is, when present, variable according to the size, location, number and stage of the parasitic cysts. This fact makes serology alone an unreliable diagnostic tool for hydatidiasis, which can frequently lead to misdiagnosis even when the diagnostic process is integrated with imaging exams. The cystic barrier also justifies the absence of available biomarkers that can be easily assessed in biological samples such as blood or urine: because humans are dead-end hosts for this parasitic disease and are infected with the meta-cestode asexual stage of the parasite, no eggs or worms are present in these biological specimens [3]. Imaging techniques are the main diagnostic tools for human cystic echinococcosis. Additionally, a molecular confirmation through PCR on cystic specimens from interventional procedures can help also in the confirmation of species involved in the infection, in cases in which taxonomic features are not sufficiently clear [3, 9].

Vascular Complications in Hydatidosis

In cases in which the *Echinococcus* spp. eggs pass the two major filters, specifically the liver and lungs, cysts can develop in other organs. This event occurs in 15% of patients. The cardiovascular system is among the possible alternative sites for the development of cysts. According to our recent review of literature of cases of aneurysms in patients with hydatidosis, arterial damage occurred at a younger age if compared to the >65 years age reference used for abdominal aortic aneurysm screening programmes [11, 12]. Among all reviewed cases, a pseudoaneurysm occurring in paediatric age was described in a 12-year-old girl diagnosed with an hydatid cyst infiltrating the abdominal aortic wall, causing the formation of a voluminous (62 mm) abdominal aortic pseudoaneurysm [12, 13].

More than one hypothesis were suggested to explain the occurrence of arterial damage in patients with hydatidosis [12]. Among these we can list:

- The development of a primary intramural form of the hydatid cyst in the vessel's wall [13–15];
- the spontaneous or surgical rupture of a hydatid cyst into an adjacent vessel, including the direct invasion from a retroperitoneal disease or from a lung lesions [16–18];
- the erosion of the arterial wall of the aorta from adjacent organs or vertebral lesions, by scolex passing into the vasa vasorum through an intimal defect lesions [11–13, 16].

The pathophysiological mechanisms leading to different kinds of arterial damage or to vascular lesions of surgical interest in patients with echinococcosis were reported in Fig. 3.1. Additionally, a pictorial summary of these mechanisms follows, in Fig. 3.2.

Among the previously published case reports and according to our recent review of these cases in literature, the clinical presentation of vascular involvement in echinococcosis could be acute [14, 17], subacute (10 days) [12, 16] or chronic (including an acute-on-chronic presentation) [13, 15, 18–21]. Chronic pain referred to the thorax and abdomen was the most frequently reported symptom at presentation [13, 15, 19–21]. In chronic patients, additional findings to the vascular lesion could be reported. Vertebral erosion in patients with hydatid cyst was occasionally described

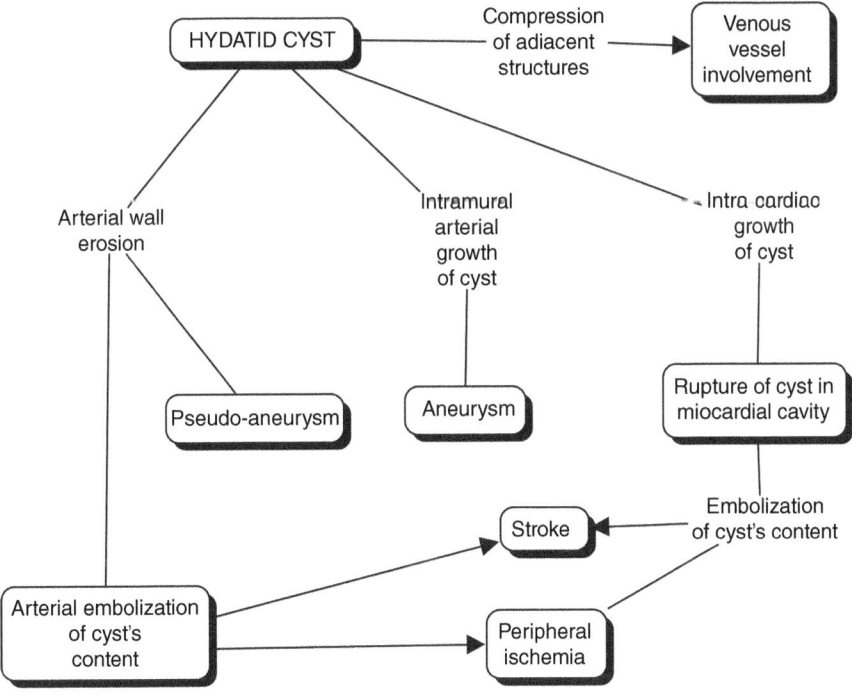

Fig. 3.1 Pathophysiology of arterial damage in Echinococcosis

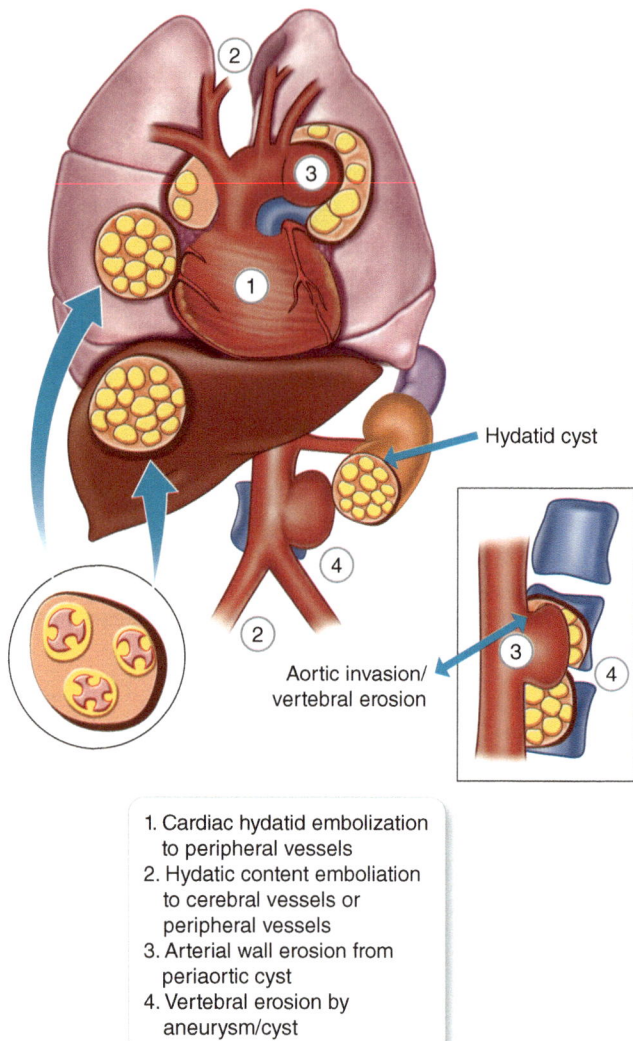

Hydatid cyst

**Aortic invasion/
vertebral erosion**

1. Cardiac hydatid embolization
   to peripheral vessels
2. Hydatic content emboliation
   to cerebral vessels or
   peripheral vessels
3. Arterial wall erosion from
   periaortic cyst
4. Vertebral erosion by
   aneurysm/cyst

Fig. 3.2 Pathophysiology of arterial damage in echinococcosis. A pictorial view. In (1) and (2). Cardiac embolization of the hydatid cyst may occur, the hydatid cyst component may reach cerebrovascular districts or peripheral vessels, leading to stroke or acute limb ischemia. (3) Arterial wall erosion by hydatid cyst can lead to the formation of pseudo-aneurysms. (4) Both the aneurysms or the hydatid can lead to vertebral erosion. The figure was adapted from the original by Valeria Silvestri, published in: Silvestri V, Mushi V, Mshana MI, Bonaventure WM, Justine N, Kihwele J, et al. Aortic aneurysm lesions in Echinococcus infection. A review of cases in literature. Vol. 50, Travel Medicine and Infectious Disease. Elsevier Ltd.; 2022. p. 102476. [12] Copyright (2022), with permission from Elsevier

[19–21]. In one case of systemic hydatidosis diagnosed in a patient with recurrent distal aortic aneurysm complicating a previous aorto-aortic graft, the concomitant vertebrae erosion was associated with history of motor deficit of lower limbs and ataxia, in addition to the chronic pain referred at presentation [19].

In those cases that manifested acutely, bleeding, neurological symptoms and limb ischemia were described as main symptoms at presentation. Bleeding occurred in the case of a 30-year-old man described by Nel et al., the patient was hospitalized for a life-threatening haemoptysis that had followed some chronic minor bleeding episodes from a periaortic hydatid pulmonary mass eroding a thoracic pseudoaneurysm [18].

Among neurological symptoms, acute headache and speech disturbance due to a huge periaortic mass infiltrating the ascending aorta and proximal arch were described in a 54-year-old lady [17].

Finally, acute limb ischemia could complicate aneurysm lesions in patients with hydatidosis. Reports of the involvement of vessels in hydatidosis include those of embolism of the germinative membranes caused by ruptured cardiac hydatid cysts. It was the case of an acute lower limb ischemia from the wall of a pseudoaneurysm of the descending thoracic aorta described by Dar et al. [14].

Cardiac Hydatidosis

Cardiac hydatid cysts are extremely rare and account for only 0.02–2% of all reported cases of hydatidosis [8, 22]. In the cardiovascular system, the heart is the most frequently affected site, harbouring 0.5–2.0% of all hydatid cysts. Echinococcus spp. larvae can enter the myocardium through the pulmonary veins, lymphatic vessels or coronary arteries [8, 22]. In some cases, myocardial invasion can occur after the rupture of a pulmonary hydatid cyst [8]. Because of the greater myocardial mass and it's volume of blood supply, the left ventricle is the site most frequently affected by cysts invasion; occasionally, the interventricular septum, the right ventricle and the pericardium may also be reached [8, 14, 22]. The signs and symptoms of cardiac hydatid cysts vary greatly depending on their location, size, and compression effects on adjacent structures ranging from an asymptomatic presentation to generating precordial discomfort, cardio palm, dyspnoea and arrhythmia. In some cases, severe life-threatening complications such as cyst rupture can occur, which can lead to acute pericarditis or cardiac tamponade, anaphylactic shock, pulmonary embolism, acute pulmonary hypertension and systemic embolization [22]. Sudden death may also occur in extreme cases [8]. Symptoms can be explained by the stretch of pericardium and the compression of coronary vessels [8].

Recently, a review of case series in literature of cases with cardiac hydatid disease was published by Banisefid et al. The authors retrieved 37 cases. Summarizing their findings, cardiac cystic echinococcosis can be secondary to other site infections, such as the lung, liver and spleen, but isolated cardiac involvement is also documented. The most commonly reported symptoms are chest pain, dyspnoea and palpitation, and normal sinus rhythm was the most common declared ECG feature.

Regarding the laboratory findings, serological tests such as *Echinococcus* indirect haemagglutination and enzyme-linked immunosorbent assay, as well as eosinophilia, were the most commonly reported findings.

Vena Cava and Lymphatic System Involvement

Venous vessels involvement was described in previous cases of hydatidosis. This can occur as a result of the venous vessel's contiguity with the structures that are involved by the cysts. Apaydin et al. reported a case of primary a mediastinal hydatid cyst which invaded the ascending aorta and the aortic arch and which extended inferior-posteriorly medial to the superior vena cava. In this case, the cava displacement was not associated with venous wall infiltration, as occurred in the aortic vessel causing pseudo-aneurysm formation [17].

Differently from *Echinococcus granulosous* infection, in which compression or rupture of cysts in the near anatomic structures is at the base of tissue involvement, in the case of *Echinococcus alveolaris,* the anatomic structures are reached and affected by lymphatic erosion, spread by lymph node metastasis [23]. Venous involvement was described to occur during this phase. *Echynococcus alveolaris* that metastasizes through the blood or lymph nodes leads to an invasive growth pattern known as "carcinoma". The enlarged lymph nodes can be located in proximity with the inferior vena cava, potentially involving this major venous vessel, in addition to the aorta or the vertebral bodies [23]. Concerning this, Xu et al. reported on a case of hepatic alveolar echinococcosis with suspected lymph node metastasis to the inferior vena cava-para-abdominal aorta. The patient underwent "middle liver resection, enlarged lymphadenectomy and inferior vena cava repair" [23].

Aortic Involvement

Aortic aneurysms have been reported in patients with hydatidosis [13–15, 17, 19–21], in which the arterial wall was described as an exceptional localization of cysts or in which the aortic involvement was associated with periaortic hydatid lesions eroding the aorta, which could be mediastinal [15–17], vertebral [20, 21] or pulmonary [18].

Available data are limited to sporadic case reports in literature [12]. According to the review of cases published in literature, the descendent thoracic aorta was the most frequently involved aortic segment [12, 14–16, 18, 20, 21]. Ascendant aorta and arch [17] and abdominal aorta were also involved [13].

In one patient, the lesion consisted of a recurrent distal aneurysm on previous aorto-aortic graft [19]. In this case, described by Volpe, the previous aortic surgery was performed for an hydatid aneurysm, which then recurred together with hydatid cyst, likely because the cyst was not removed entirely during the first procedure [19]. The aorta remodelling with concomitant aneurysm re-expansion was also observed after the endovascular treatment of the recurrent aneurysm [19].

Occasionally, an additional challenge reported in the case of aneurysms located in the aortic arch and in descendent thoracic aorta was the contiguity with vena cava, leading to distortion of its structure [15, 17].

Among other complications, an acute limb ischemia could occur in patients diagnosed with aneurysms in Echinococcosis. In a case described by Dar et al., an acute limb ischemia was the first sign at clinical presentation of a lower descending aortic pseudo-aneurysm. Ischemia was secondary to an aortic pseudo-aneurysm occurring in the lower descending thoracic aorta with multiple small cysts in its cavity. The pseudoaneurysm was communicating with the aorta through a small rent in the wall of the aorta [14].

Findings from our recent review of cases of aortic involvement in hydatidiasis are summarized in Table 3.1, previously published in the original paper: *Silvestri V, Mushi V, Mshana MI, Bonaventure WM, Justine N, Kihwele J,* et al. *Aortic aneurysm lesions in Echinococcus infection. A review of cases in literature. Vol. 50, Travel Medicine and Infectious Disease. Elsevier Ltd; 2022. p. 102476* (Table 3.1).

Diagnostic Management for Cases of Vascular Interest

In those cases with an indication for surgical treatment, including cases of vascular surgical interest, a preoperative serologic tests for *Echinococcus* spp. (including reaction to passive haemagglutination, immunofluorescence assay and enzyme-linked immunosorbent assay) should be performed when patients are from known endemic areas [19–21], even though, as observed in the introduction, results have a rate of false negatives due to the barrier exerted by the cyst structure, which isolates the parasite antigens from the systemic circulation, and can be negative in up to 50% especially in case of extra-pulmonary hydatid disease [12, 13].

Because of the diagnostic limit of serology, imaging studies should be integrated in the diagnostic flow. Ultrasound imaging has better sensitivity than serological testing for detecting cardiac, liver and non-hepatic Echinococcosis, especially when combined with other modalities such as CT and/or magnetic resonance imaging [24]. In the case of cardiac echinococcosis, transthoracic echocardiography is sensitive and specific in detecting cardiac cysts [8, 22].

Imaging tools like CT and MRI can complement ultrasound diagnostics, by showing the exact anatomical location of the aneurysm sac and the nature of the internal and external structures of an associated hydatid cyst [19]. These advanced imaging tools can quantify the extension of hydatid cysts [22]. In cases of cardiac involvement by hydatid cyst, MRI can clearly demonstrate the exact location in cardiac structures and define its relationship with adjacent structures. On T1-weighted images, the hydatid cyst can be observed as an hypointense lesion, while on T2-weighted images, the lesion appears hyperintense, with a low-signal intensity rim representing the peri cyst structure [22]. MRI is also the technique used for post-treatment follow-up in surgically managed cases [14].

Differently from MRI, CT scan is the greatest tool for displaying the calcification of the cyst wall [22].

Table 3.1 Aortic damage in Echinococcosis: cases in literature

Author/year	Age	Sex	Comorbidities	Symptoms and signs	Echinococcus details	Vascular findings	Surgical treatment	Pharmacological treatment	Outcome
Biglioli 1995	43	M	n.s	Subacute Toraco-lumbar pain (10 days)	Surgical finding of peri-aortic daughter cysts	Descending thoracic aorta posterior aneurysm communicating with periaortic hydatic cyst	Thoracic aortic patch and cyst removal	No anti-parasitic treatment	Uneventful 2 years follow up
Zachariev 1997	44	M	Chronic hypertension	Chronic subcostal arch pain	Surgical finding of periaortic mass with scolices	Descending thoracic aorta false aneurysm (150 mm) on chronic dissection and vertebral erosion	Aortic aneurysm resection, hydatid cyst sterilization and aorto-aortic graft (dacron)	Post-operatory mebendazole (1 year)	Uneventful
Posacioglu 1999	48	F	n.s.	Chronic chest pain (6 months)	Positive serology. Surgical finding of intramural aortic hydatid cyst	Descending aortic pseudo-aneurysm (80 cm × 50 mm) and inferior vena cava and right atrium compression	Aortic aneurysm resection, hydatid cyst resection and aorto-aortic graft (dacron)	Post-operatory mebendazole	Uneventful 3 month follow up
Nel 2001	38	M	Smoke	Chronic haemoptysis (6 months) Pleuritic chest pain (2 weeks)	Surgical finding of hydatid cyst eroding aorta	Descending thoracic aorta small saccular aneurysm (60 mm) and periaortic eroding lung mass	Aortic aneurysm resection, hydatid cyst excision, aorto-aortic graft (polyester) and lung lower-lobe lobectomy	Post-operatory albendazole	Uneventful 6 months follow up

Author/Year	Age	Sex	History	Symptoms	Diagnosis/Finding	Aneurysm	Treatment	Post-operative	Outcome
Pulathan 2004	12	F	n.s.	Chronic abdominal pain (1 month)	Negative serology Surgical finding of hydatid cyst in aortic wall	Abdominal aortic pseudoaneurysm (62 mm)	Aorto-iliac aneurysm resection, hydatid cyst excision, aortoiliac by-pass and cross-over (PTFE)	Post-operatory albendazole (1 month)	Uneventful 1 year follow up
Volpe 2006	51	M	Descending thoracic aorta bypass for hydatid aneurysm	Chronic thoraco-abdominal pain, lower limbs motor deficit, ataxia	Surgical finding of aortic wall hydatid cyst (previous diagnosis)	Recurrent descending thoracic aorta Saccular aneurysm and vertebral erosion	Custom-made endovascular repair	No antiparasitic treatment	Stenting of distal graft end-point stenosis required. Vertebral stabilization for erosion. Residual paraplegia and Permanent bladder catheter
Apaydin 2007	54	F	Abdominal aortic aneurysm (incidental finding)	Acute Headache, Speech disturbance	Aortic hydatid cyst On surgical specimen	Ascending aorta and proximal arch periaortic infiltrating mass (80 mm); superior vena cava and right pulmonary artery displacement	Ascending aorta and arch resection; hydatid cyst excision; T graft reconstruction (dacron)	Post-operatory albendazole (1 year)	Uneventful

(continued)

Table 3.1 (continued)

Author/year	Age	Sex	Comorbidities	Symptoms and signs	Echinococcus details	Vascular findings	Surgical treatment	Pharmacological treatment	Outcome
Dar 2010	45	F	n.s.	Acute lower limb ischemia (1 day)	Positive serology Surgical finding of aortic hydatid cyst	Descending thoracic aorta pseudo-aneurysm	Pseudoaneurysm excision and aortorrhaphies	n.s.	Uneventful 6 month follow up
Mozafar 2020	40	M	Rheumatoid arthritis	Chronic back pain (4 months)	Positive fine needle aspiration	Descending thoracic aorta saccular aneurysm (60 mm) and vertebral erosion	Endovascular Aneurysm Repair (EVAR)	Albendazole 4 years after first surgical treatment	Vertebral erosion but intact endograft at follow-up

Reprinted from: Silvestri V, Mushi V, Mshana MI, Bonaventure WM, Justine N, Kihwele J, et al. Aortic aneurysm lesions in Echinococcus infection. A review of cases in literature. Vol. 50, Travel Medicine and Infectious Disease. Elsevier Ltd; 2022. p. 102476. [12] Copyright (2022), with permission from Elsevier

Finally, an angiography study can define the communication between the aortic lumen and the cyst [19] and can offer treatment options in those diagnosed cases that can be converted to an endovascular interventional approach.

Surgical Management

Because of the rarity of these lesions, no standard surgical technique is currently recommended [12]. In the lack of general guidelines, in aneurysm cases, the indication for surgery is usually based on the risk of aneurysm rupture. Additionally, the surgical plan should consider the need to avoid the distal hydatid cyst migration. The concomitant complete surgical removal of the cysts and of its capsule, which characterize echinococcosis, is considered an essential action to prevent potentially fatal cyst rupture and to avoid the risk of recurring disease [12, 24]. In previous cases in which no radical removal of cysts from the surgical field was achieved, the recurrence of both the aneurysm and cyst was described to occur after a first major vascular intervention, as described by Volpe et al. [19]. In their case, the aorta remodelling with concomitant aneurysm re-expansion was observed not only after the first open surgery for aortic aneurysms in echinococcosis but also after the endovascular treatment of the recurrent aneurysm with cyst re-expansion [19]. This case suggests that the endovascular treatment, by necessarily leaving in site the *Echinococcus* cysts, can provide a temporary solution but not be a first-choice strategy for radical treatment.

For the cases with cardiac involvement, it was discussed previously that embolic complications can occur if the cyst breaks into myocardial cavity and if its content embolizes systemically. When this occurs, life-threatening complications in the form of acute pericarditis or cardiac tamponade, anaphylactic shock, pulmonary embolism, acute pulmonary hypertension and systemic embolization can occur [22]. The acknowledgement of this risk seams to guide the surgical strategy. In case of cardiac involvement, even for asymptomatic patients, surgical excision under cardiopulmonary bypass is still required for the management of cardiac hydatidosis [22]. According to the recent review of cases in literature of cardiac hydatidosis by Banisefid et al., a combination of surgical methods and pharmacological management was reported in the majority of cases, which were associated with appropriate outcomes, so the rates of mortality and recurrence were not considerable [8]. The pharmacological treatment of choice is albendazole. This management has yielded high success rates. Proto-scolicidal agents such as iodine, hypertonic saline, methylene blue or ethanol can be used to sterilize hydatid cysts prior to enucleation and pericardial cavity irrigation, still none of these agents are completely safe and effective for intraoperative usage [22].

We have seen that venous vessels, vena cava *in primis*, can be affected by the cyst invasion. The surgical approach used in cases with venous and lympatic involvement in alveolar hydatidosis was described once in literature and reported by Wu et al. The case concerned vena cava involvement by metastatic lymph nodes in hepatic alveolar echinococcosis and was managed with "middle liver resection, enlarged lymphadenectomy and inferior vena cava repair". The importance of following, through surgery, the principle of being tumour-free, with removal of lesions from the important structures that needed to be preserved, such as major blood vessels, was emphasized by authors as a step to prevent postoperative echinococcosis recurrence and improve the patient's quality of life. Thus, in their case, the cyst removal was followed by the inferior vena cava-para-aortic lymph nodes stripping to reach skeletonization [23].

In the cases in which the vessel involved by hydatidosis is the aorta, the aortic reconstruction with graft interposition was suggested as the treatment of choice [17]. With the risk of hydatid cyst recurrence well in mind, this technique was preferred to the aortic patch, which could reduce the aortic clamping needed to achieve the closure of the communication between the peri-cyst and aorta [16], but at potential cost of recurrent lesion requiring reintervention [19].

Even though open surgery was described in the majority of the (although rare) cases in literature, the endovascular exclusion of the systemic circulation from the hydatid mass with an endograft was described as a bridge treatment to open surgery, to reduce the risk of vessel rupture, anaphylactic shock and systemic dissemination of disease caused by the rupture of the mother cyst [12, 19]. The endovascular treatment, in cases in which the lesion is anatomically suitable for this approach, could suit patients in whom a complete surgical resection is at high risk for systemic dissemination of the disease. Non-invasive approach could also be an option for palliative care [12, 19].

Among the examples in literature of an endovascular approach to treat vascular lesions in patients with hydatidosis, we can report the recurrent hydatid aneurysm on a previous descending thoracic patch complicated by vertebral erosion, motor deficit of lower limbs and ataxia, described by Volpe et al. and discussed earlier. In this case, the endovascular treatment was the best option for hydatid complications occurring in a patient with previous aortic surgery, and the implant of an endograft allowed a protection against fistulisation and embolization of the disease. Notwithstanding treatment, cyst and aneurysm recurrence occurred after the first endovascular procedure, emphasizing how the radical removal of cyst is important to prevent, together with echinococcosis relapse, the recurrence of the arterial lesion [19].

Endovascular approach was also indicated to treat a challenging aneurysm lesion involving the descendent thoracic aorta in a 40-year-old patient, which was complicated with vertebral erosion [21]. Even though the endovascular treatment allows the exclusion of the aneurysm lesion, it should be emphasized that this approach can't solve the local compressive effects of the hydatid mass, nor its progressive invasion, and the accurate surgical resection of the mother cyst remains critical to avoid systemic dissemination [12, 17, 19].

Because the incomplete removal of hydatid cyst from the surgical field can cause recurrence of the disease, regardless of the surgical technique used, a close followup of treated patients is warranted to detect possible recurrence at an early stage [12, 14, 17]. Antiparasitic drug therapy (albendazole or mebenzazole) should also be considered to minimize the risk of hydatidiasis relapse after surgical treatment

[13–15, 17, 18, 20, 24]. Protracting albendazole treatment for 6 months was suggested by some authors as an appropriate treatment length [24].

Finally, not all cases are suitable for surgical treatment. It should always be kept in mind that medical therapy alone should be considered in cases unsuitable for surgery [12, 22].

Conclusion

Cardiovascular system can be involved by *Echinococcus* spp. infection, mainly in the form of aortic aneurysm. Hydatid disease should be considered as an uncommon differential diagnosis in patients with saccular aneurysms of the aorta that are resident, originating or travelling in endemic areas. A high suspicion for diagnosis together with a specific approach for surgical intervention is needed to correctly detect the affected patients, to successfully treat the vascular lesion but also to accurately remove the associated hydatid disease, preventing the recurrence of the parasitic disease and, together with it, of the vascular condition. The follow-up of surgical treated patients is essential to promptly detect any recurrent lesions of hydatidiasis and to improve the patient's outcome.

The exact prevalence of vascular lesions as co-occurring conditions in patients with hydatidosis is unknown, but it is likely to be underestimated due to the lack of registers in endemic areas. Exploratory population-based studies combining vascular and parasitological assessment in endemic settings could be useful to fill this gap, providing good-quality data that will better inform us on these specific non-communicable diseases of parasitological interest, in accordance with the newly launched revised WHO 2021–2030 NTD Roadmap, which aims at the elimination of morbidity related to non-communicable diseases in all endemic countries by 2030 [25].

References

1. Khan MB, Sonaimuthu P, Lau YL, Al-mekhlafi HM, Mahmud R, Kavana N, et al. High seroprevalence of echinococossis , schistosomiasis and toxoplasmosis among the populations in Babati and Monduli districts, Tanzania. Parasit Vectors. 2014:1–9.
2. WHO. Neglected Tropical Diseases. 2023. Available from: https://www.who.int/news-room/questions-and-answers/item/neglected-tropical-diseases
3. Casulli A, Abela-Ridder B, Petrone D, Fabiani M, Bobić B, Carmena D, et al. Unveiling the incidences and trends of the neglected zoonosis cystic echinococcosis in Europe: a systematic review from the MEmE project. Lancet Infect Dis. 2023;23(3):e95–107.
4. Fornaciari A, Gaeta R, Cavallini L, Aringhieri G, Ishak R, Bruschi F, et al. A 13th-century cystic echinococcosis from the cemetery of the monastery of Badia Pozzeveri (Lucca, Italy). Int J Paleopathol. 2020;31:79–88. https://doi.org/10.1016/j.ijpp.2020.10.005.
5. Mowlavi G, Kacki S, Dupouy-Camet J, Mobedi I, Makki M, Harandi MF, et al. Probable hepatic capillariosis and hydatidosis in an adolescent from the late Roman period buried in Amiens (France). Parasite. 2014;21:9.

6. Gaeta R, Giuffra V. Disseminated cystic echinococcosis of Ferdinando II de' Medici, Grand Duke of Tuscany (1610–1670). J Infect. 2019;79(5):462–70.

7. Wen H, Vuitton L, Tuxun T, Li J, Vuitton DA, Zhang WMD. Echinococcosis: advances in the 21st Century. Clin Microbiol Rev. 2019;32(2):e00075–18.

8. Banisefid E, Baghernezhad K, Beheshti R, Hamzehzadeh S, Nemati S, Samadifar Z, et al. Cardiac hydatid disease; a systematic review. BMC Infect Dis. 2023;23(1):1–17.

9. Regan S, Triant VA, Perez J, Regan S, Massaro JM, Meigs JB, Grinspoon SKDRS, Regan S. Cardiovascular risk prediction functions underestimate risk in HIV infection. Circulation. 2018;21(137):2203–14.

10. Khalili N, Iranpour P, Khalili N, Haseli S. Hydatid disease: a pictorial review of uncommon locations. Iran J Med Sci. 2023;48(2):118–29.

11. Sakalihasan N, Michel JB, Katsargyris A, Kuivaniemi H, Defraigne JO, Nchimi A, Powell JT, Yoshimura KHR. Abdominal aortic aneurysms. Nat Rev Dis Prim. 2018;4(1):34.

12. Silvestri V, Mushi V, Mshana MI, Bonaventure WM, Justine N, Kihwele J, et al. Aortic aneurysm lesions in Echinococcus infection. A review of cases in literature. Travel Med Infect Dis. 2022;50:102476.

13. Pulathan Z, Cay A, Güven YSH. Hydatid cyst of the abdominal aorta and common iliac arteries complicated by a false aneurysm: a case report. J Paediatr Surg. 2004;39(4):637–9.

14. Dar AM. Hydatid embolism from a thoracic aortic pseudoaneurysm presenting as gangrenous toes. Gen Thorac Cardiovasc Surg. 2010:344–7.

15. Posacioglu H, Bakalim T, Cikirikcioglu M, Yuce G, Telli A, Posacioglu H, et al. Intramural hydatid cyst of descending aorta complicated by false aneurysm intramural hydatid cyst of descending aorta complicated by false aneurysm. Scand Cardiovasc J. 2009;7431:2–5.

16. Biglioli P, Spirito R, Roberto M, Parolari A, Agrifoglio M, Pompilio G, Arena V. False hydatic aneurysm of the thoracic aorta. Ann Thorac Surg. 1995;4975(94):5–6.

17. Apaydin AZ, Oguz E, Zoghi M. Hydatid cyst involving the aortic arch. Eur J Cardiothorac Surg. 2007;31:2006–8.

18. Nel JD, Kriegler SG, Van Vuuren WM, Harris DGBC. An unusual cause of nearly fatal hemoptysis. Respiration. 2001;7505:635–6.

19. Volpe P, Dalainas I, Ruggieri M, Nano G, Paroni G, Rotondo G. Endovascular treatment of the descending thoracic aorta in a patient with a hydatid pseudoaneurysm. J Vasc Surg. 2006:2000–3.

20. Zakhariev T, Stankev M, Baev B, Iliev R, Tschirkov A. A rare case of hydatid cyst perrceived as false aneurysm of thoracic aorta. J Thorac Cardiovasc Surg. 1997;113(4):792–3.

21. Mozafar M, Haghighatkhah H, Khoshnoud RJ, Zarrintan S, Rakhshani N. Saccular mycotic aneurysm of descending thoracic aorta secondary to vertebral hydatid disease: a rare case. 2021:1–6.

22. Alvi MA, Ali RMA, Khan S, Saqib M, Qamar W, Li L, et al. Past and present of diagnosis of echinococcosis: a review (1999–2021). Acta Trop. 2023;243:106925.

23. Xu X, Gao C, Qian X, Liu H, Wang Z, Zhou H, et al. Treatment of complicated hepatic alveolar echinococcosis disease with suspicious lymph node remote metastasis near the inferior vena cava-abdominal aorta: a case report and literature review. Front Oncol. 2022;12:1–8.

24. Wedin JO, Astudillo RM, Kurland S, Grinnemo K-H, Astudillo R, Vikholm P, et al. A rare case of cardiac echinococcosis: the role of multimodality imaging. CASE. 2021;5(4):230–4.

25. Ending the neglect to attain the Sustainable Development Goals: a strategic framework for integrated control and management of skin-related neglected tropical diseases. Geneva: World Health Organization; 2022. Available at https://www.who.int/publications/i/item/9789240010352.

Amoebiasis

4

Contents

Introduction

Entamoeba species are endobiotic amoebae-colonizing animal species which have evolved with humans since antiquity. These protozoal parasites have a two-stage life cycle, with an environmental infectious cyst and a dividing trophozoite residing in the human intestine [1]. At least eight species of *Entamoeba* have the ability to infect humans primarily in the intestinal tract [2]., where they divide and encyst. Most *Entamoeba* infections in humans appear to be caused by non-pathogenic species, for example, *Entamoeba dispar* and *Entamoeba coli*. Among all *Entamoeba* spp., *Entamoeba histolytica* is the only one that can express virulence in human. As

© The Author(s), under exclusive license to Springer Nature   49
Switzerland AG 2024
V. Silvestri et al., *Vascular Damage in Neglected Tropical Diseases*,
https://doi.org/10.1007/978-3-031-53353-2_4

the causative agent of amoebiasis, it is responsible for dysentery and liver abscesses [1].

Amoebic colitis has been known since antiquity. *Entamoeba histolytica* (*E. histolytica*) was observed by paleo pathologists through the study of parasite markers from preserved ancient faeces (coprolites) or from sediment samples taken from those contexts that potentially contain human faecal matter [3]. Written documents also suggest that the disease was known in the past. Together with other diseases of parasitological interest, such as enteric helminthiasis or pulmonary hydatid disease, Hippocrates described cases of hepatic lesions following protracted diarrhoea that are reminiscent of amebiasis [4] as *"Dysenteries, [that] when they set in with fever, alvine discharges of a mixed character, or with inflammation of the liver … are bad"*. The parasite responsible of the disease was identified during the XIX century, in 1875, by the Russian physician Fedor Aleksandrovich Lösch, who observed trophozoites of the amoeba protozoa in the stool and colonic ulcerations [5, 6]. In 1883, Koch demonstrated that there were amoebae in the sections of a human ulcerated bowel, demonstrating the connection between the parasite and the intestinal lesion [7].

Even though *Entamoeba* is not listed among the WHO Neglected Tropical Diseases, it was previously emphasized by Editors of PLOS that the community of NTD investigators conduct research and public health efforts on an expanded group of conditions that constitute chronic and debilitating conditions disproportionately affecting populations living in extreme poverty, which complies with the definition of NTD [8]. Because of the description of vascular damage in patients with amoebiasis, and its suitability for the inclusion into this wider list of neglected conditions, we dedicated one chapter of this book to this protozoal infestation.

Epidemiology

E. histolytica is a globally distributed protozoan parasite, prevalent in countries with poor sanitation [9]. Its distribution is favoured by the lack of personal hygiene, by the use of stagnant water, the lack of sanitary disposal system, the use of human faeces in agriculture and by the intense fly breeding [10]. The predisposing environmental conditions of lack of access to clean water and inadequate improved sanitation are a condition that was estimated to involve 780 million and 2.5 billion people, respectively [2, 10].

Tropical and subtropical regions such as Central and South America, Asia and Africa. Bangladesh, India, Brazil, Colombia, Mexico and China are on the top list of most affected countries [10]. Even though the genus *Entamoeba* consists of at least eight species (*E. bangladeshi, E. coli, E. dispar, E. gingivalis, E. hartmanni, E. histolytica, E. moshkovskii* and *E. polecki*) that are able to inhabit in the human intestine, *E. histolytica* is the unique species that is pathogenic to human. The infection is mainly transmitted via ingestion of water or food contaminated by faeces containing *E. histolytica* cysts, which are resistant to disinfection and can survive in suitable aquatic environments for several months [2].

Amoebiasis is the third potentially deadly parasitic disease, after malaria and schistosomiasis [2]. Together with other protozoal infections such as *Cryptosporidium spp* and *Giardia intestinalis*, amoebiasis is a cause of significant gastrointestinal morbidity, malnutrition and mortality worldwide. According to the Global Burden of Disease Study, in 2010, *Entamoeba histolytica* was responsible for 2.2 million disability-adjusted life years (DALYs), while its annual mortality was estimated at 100,000 cases [2].

When analysing amoebiasis in the context of different continents through extensive examination, a prevalence of the condition reaching 12.4% was observed from different African settings. The prevalence of extraintestinal amoebiasis due to *E. histolytica* assessed by serology was even higher, and it was estimated at 15–70%. These findings were likely to be due to hygienic and environmental conditions [10]. In Asia, the infection is mainly reported in South-Eastern regions where the poor hygienic conditions, the release of human faeces in the environment and the lack of an effective sewage system encourage its spread. The political instability of some territories such as the Gaza Strip, leading to poverty, poor personal hygiene, lack of access to safe water and inefficiency of health systems could be responsible for the prevalence of 70% observed in this area [10]. In North America, the immigration and travels from endemic areas have led to the emergence of amoebiasis in these developed countries, where in 2007, 411 cases of intestinal disease due to *E. histolytica* were reported in California with an estimated prevalence of nearly 4%, while in Mexico, amoebiasis ranked among the 20 most common causes of death, with a prevalence of 42% [10]. Amoebiasis is endemic in South America, particularly in Brazil, Ecuador and Colombia. In Brazil, intestinal amoebiasis due to *E. histolytica* was prevalent in 1% of analysed cases [10]. The disease is also present in Australia, particularly in northern districts, principally occurring in indigenous people or among immigrants or travellers returning from endemic countries [10]. In Europe, amoebiasis is a public health issue introduced mainly from other endemic foci. At present, all clinical forms of amoebiasis have been increasing in incidence due to immigration from endemic regions and a growing of tourists travelling to European countries [10].

Pathophysiology

Entamoeba histolytica has a two-stage life cycle, with an environmental infectious cyst and a dividing trophozoite residing in the human intestine [1]. Approximately 90% of infected individuals are asymptomatic carriers of the disease [2]. Even though the host maintains the parasite under control while it is living in the intestinal lumen and feeding on bacteria, 1% of infected individuals develop the invasive form [2]. Due to unknown signals, *E. histolytica* can lead to the symptomatic infection, which can have different degrees of severity. A clinically symptomatic infection causes intestinal amoebiasis, an inflammatory dysentery characterized by the destruction of muco-epithelial barrier, the overproduction of mucus, the killing of host cells through necrosis or apoptotic processes [1, 7]. During the invasion stage, the amoebae released from the cysts adhere to the mucus layer of the colon through the interaction between the parasites' surface lectin molecules and the host correspondent protein and with residues of mucin oligosaccharides. In this way, *E. histolytica* subverts the physical and chemical barrier constituted by intestinal mucous, by secreting glycosidases that cleave the lateral sugar residues of mucin, cysteine proteases and other antimicrobial molecules [7]. In symptomatic cases, the parasite invades the mucosa and intestinal tissue, feeding on phagocytosed erythrocytes and apoptotic and necrotic cells, while those products that are released by amoebae can bind to the epithelial intercellular junctions, interrupting them and causing a downregulation of cell-cell adhesion molecules [7]. Trophozoites may then disseminate through the portal vein system and invade the liver where it forms abscesses [1].

Amoebic colitis clinical manifestations can be intestinal and extra-intestinal. They share several common symptoms, such as fever, loss of appetite or nausea [2]. The pathology changes can range from mucosal thickening; multiple discrete ulcers separated by regions of colonic mucosa of normal appearance; diffusely inflamed and oedematous mucosa; and necrosis and perforation of the intestinal wall, which can mimic inflammatory bowel disease [5, 6]. The symptoms that characterize intestinal amoebiasis range from abdominal pain and ulcerative colitis with mucous and blood (amoebic dysentery) to appendicitis and ulcers (ameboma). Occasionally, the parasites can reach the liver through the portal vein, and they can cause one of the main extraintestinal infections, which is amoebic liver abscess. Additionally, other extraintestinal sites can be reached, such as the lungs and brain, mainly in immunocompromised patients. Both intestinal and extraintestinal manifestations of amoebiasis can be fatal if left untreated [6].

As for the case of hepatic involvement in amoebiasis, liver abscess is known to occur in 3–9% of all cases [11], and from months to years after travel or residency in an endemic area [5]. An estimated 40,000–100,000 people die yearly from amoebic liver abscess, prevalently affecting men between the age of 18 and 50, which bear rates 3–20 times higher than other populations, likely because of hormonal effects or alcohol assumption [5, 6]. Complications of liver abscess could also not be limited to the hepatic region: thoracic empyema or acute peritonitis has also been occasionally described [11]. In many of these cases of extra-intestinal manifestations, no bowel symptoms can be observed, and stool microscopy can be negative for both *E. histolytica* trophozoites and cysts [5]. The false-negative results of classical laboratory investigations challenge the diagnosis of these conditions [6].

Diagnosis

The clinical diagnosis of amoebiasis is rather difficult due to poor knowledge of the clinicians in non-endemic regions or because of the non-specific nature of the symptoms [10]. Laboratory diagnostic methods of amoebiasis are mainly based on parasitological investigations including microscopy and culture, which is considered the gold standard. Serological tests such as enzyme-linked immunosorbent assay, indirect haemagglutination, latex agglutination, or molecular techniques are also available. In extraintestinal amoebiasis, the stool examination has a low sensitivity against serological methods, while in recent decades, polymerase chain reaction (PCR)-based techniques have improved their sensibility. Imaging methods such as radiography, computed tomography (CT), magnetic resonance imaging (MRI) or ultrasonography can be helpful in the diagnostic workflow for accurate diagnosis of intestinal and extraintestinal amoebiasis [2].

Vascular Complications in Amoebiasis

Pathophysiological Mechanisms

As we have emphasized in the previous chapters, *E. histolytica* has cytolytic capabilities which are well documented in intestinal tissues [7, 9]. Minutes after contact with amoebic trophozoites, human cells become immobile, and they lose their cytoplasmic granules, their structures and nucleus. Amoebic pores are responsible for the cytolysis induced by the parasite. These pores are assembled with peptides in lipid bilayers, which are structurally related to granulins and NK-lysins produced by mammalian T-cells. But cytolysis is not the only mechanism for host invasion. An additional strategy is the direct enzymatic digestion of extracellular matrix proteins of the invaded tissue, through cysteine proteinases. A third mechanism of invasion is the direct induction of apoptosis of mammalian cells by *E. histolytica* trophozoites [5].

If the ones reported earlier are the mechanisms that lead to tissue invasion and damage in general, it was suggested that a direct action of trophozoites against the vessels wall could lead to the vascular extra-intestinal manifestation of the disease [9].

In the same way, vascular damage could be due to the induction of inflammation, then extended to vessels. *E. histolytica* cysteine proteinases amplify interleukin-1-mediated inflammation, by cleaving the precursor of interleukin-1 into its active mature form. The cytokines and cyclo-oxygenase response attracts neutrophils and macrophages to the site of amoebic invasion [5]. The inflammation triggered through these patterns may then lead to the inflammatory damage of the vascular wall and to an aneurysm formation [9]. In relation to the hypothesis of an inflammation-induced vascular damage, it is of interest that the co-occurrence of amoebiasis in three paediatric cases affected by Kawasaki disease, diagnosed with coronary artery aneurysm, was reported previously. It was suggested that the microorganisms might have a role in the aetiology of vasculitis leading to aneurysm formation, even though causality couldn't be ascertained [9, 12]. It is also interesting that amoebiasis could be included in the differential diagnosis for other autoimmune conditions, such as Bechet's disease: the cecal lesions, aphthae and multiple exudative erosions observed in amoebiasis could be misinterpreted as intestinal Behçet's disease, a chronic inflammatory disorder that is characterized by multiple ulcers [13], but also by potential vascular damage including aneurysms [14].

A summary of the suggested pathophysiology that could explain vascular damage observed in patients with *Entamoeba histolytica* infestation is given in Fig. 4.1.

Potential Vascular Involvement in Amoebiasis

Vascular involvement in patients with amoebiasis was described in the form of coronary artery aneurysms, infrarenal aortic aneurysms and pseudo-aneurysms in hepatic abscesses. Coronary aneurysms were diagnosed in three paediatric patients with Kawasaki disease. Given the paucity of data, no relation of causation could be determined between the two diagnoses [15]. Aortic involvement co-occurred in one case of amoebiasis (which was discussed but not included directly in a previous review from our group, because it focused on pseudo-aneurysms in hepatic amoebic abscess) [9, 16]. Pseudo-aneurysms in hepatic liver abscess are rarely described, but some information on diagnostic challenges and treatment could be assessed by the clinical reports available in the literature for this condition [9]. A summary of the available case in literature is given in Tables 4.1 and 4.2.

Aortic Involvement

One case of co-occurrent aortic involvement in a patient with amoebiasis was described in the literature (Table 4.1). In this case, surgery was performed in a 68-year-old patient for a symptomatic infrarenal aortic aneurysm of 7 × 8 cm in diameter, with an additional common iliac aneurysm of 3 × 3 cm. During clinical interview, the patient mentions an episode of amoebic dysentery which occurred while serving the US army in the Philippines, 30 years previously. During surgery, the arterial wall appeared oedematous and firmly adherent to the duodenum. The

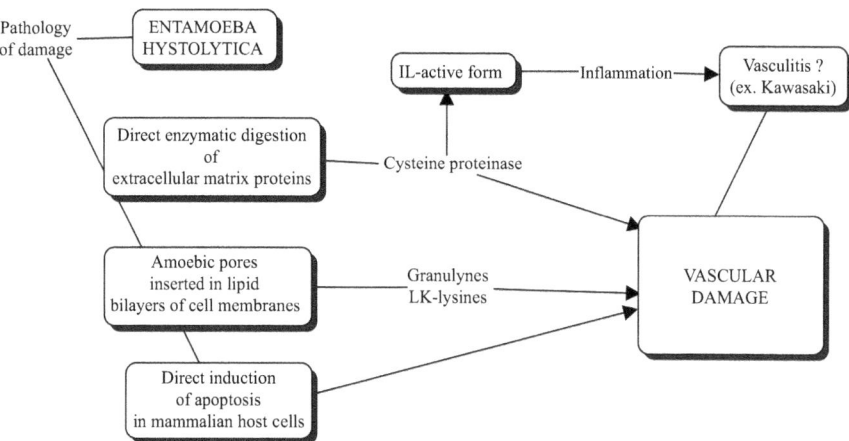

Fig. 4.1 Pathophysiology of vascular damage in Entamoeba histolytica infestation

Table 4.1 Summary of case reports of aneurysms occurring in patients with amoebiasis. Aorta and coronary artery involvement cases

Author date	Age	Sex	Clinical presentation	Abscess drainage	Vascular lesion	Pharmacological therapy	Interventional treatment	Vascular outcome
Cases of aorta involvement								
Katz 1980	68	M	History of amoebiasis 30 years previously. One day history of severe right groin pain radiating to his back, and nausea	n.a.	Infrarenal aortic (7 × 8 cm) and right common iliac aneurysm (3 × 3 cm) complicated by watery diarrhea on 3rd day after surgery	Metronidazole on 13th day post op	Aorta–bis-iliac arteries graft	No complications reported to the vascular graft by the overlapping amoebiasis
Cases of coronary artery involvement								
Viswanathan 2019	4	M	Persistent fever for 18 days; abdominal pain, hepatic abscess with positive amoebic serology	No	Proximal right coronary artery saccular aneurysm (RCA Z score 4.31), left main coronary (LMCA Z score 3.22), left anterior descending artery (LAD-Z score 2.55)	IVIG 2 g/kg; anti amoebicidal drugs; low dose Aspirin	None	Normalization of echo-cardio graphic findings in 6 months
Viswanathan 2019	5	F	Remittent fever of 7 days, redness of lips and palpable cervical lymph node. Macular rash, non-purulent congiuntivitis	Yes, at diagnosis (positive serology)	Coronary aneurysm LMCA-Z score 0.06, LAD -Z score of 1.91 and RCA -Z score of 5.97	IVIG 2 g/kg, systemic amoebicidal	Drainage of hepatic abscess	Symptoms resolved 3 days after hepatic drainage and amoebicidal therapy. Steady regression of coronary artery abnormalities in 3 months

Table 4.2 Summary of case reports of aneurysms occurring in patients with amoebiasis. Hepatic artery involvement

Author date	Age	Sex	Clinical presentation	Abscess drainage	Vascular lesion	Pharmacological therapy	Interventional treatment	Vascular outcome
Gopanpallikar 1997	40	M	Recurrent haemorrhage of upper gastrointestinal tract	n.a.	Hepatic a.aneurysm	n.a.	n.a.	n.a.
Yanagisawa 2002	51	M	Peritonitis, perforating appendicitis	13 days before vascular diagnosis	Hepatic a. aneurysm ruptured in liver abscess, with haemobilia	Metronidazole started on admission for peritonitis	Embolization	Discharged 5 weeks after procedure. Uneventful
Tacconi 2009	31	M	Anorexia; cough; left side thoracic pain (7 days)	Yes (only procedure)	Hepatic a. aneurysm	Metronidazole i.v. every 8 h. for 15 days +50 ml metronidazole intra-abscess	Hepatic abscess drainage	Aneurysm disappearance after 2 months
Priyadarshi 2019	52	M	Fever; right hypocondrium pain (20 days) Melena (2 weeks) haemobilia, anaemia, leukocytosis, liver enzimes increase	Yes (only procedure)	Right hepatic aneurysm(10 mm) + contained rupture in sub-phrenic region	Started not specified oral anti-amoebic in another hospital 1 week before admission	Hepatic abscess drainage (spontaneous aneurysm thrombosis 2 days after procedure)	Spontaneous aneurysm thrombosis after hepatic drainage, on day 2. Hepatic drainage removed after 20 days

Khan 2015	50	M	Fever, anorexia, vomiting, icterus, leukocytosis, impairment of liver function test (10 days)	Yes, 36 h before vascular diagnosis	Segmental branch of right hepatic artery aneurysm	Broad spectrum antibiotics covering gram negative bacteria + M etronidazole	Embolization	Uneventful
Yadav 2015	45	M	Abdominal pain, fever, hepatomegaly (10 days) hematemesis, melena, anemia, hematobilia (8 days after metronidazole)	Yes, on 2nd post-operatory day	Pseudoaneurysm 7th branch of hepatic a.	Metronidazole i.v. on admission	Embolization+ Hepatic abscess drainage	Complete occlusion of pseudo-aneurysm after embolization.

Reprinted from: Silvestri V, Ngasala B. Hepatic aneurysm in patients with amoebic liver abscess. A review of cases in literature. Travel Med Infect Dis. 2022 Mar–Apr; 46:102274. Copyright (2022), with permission from Elsevier

open surgery that was performed to correct the symptomatic aortic aneurysm lesion was complicated by the onset of diarrhoea on the third post-operatory day; still only 14 days after aorto-bisiliac surgery, amoebic cysts were detected in stools, allowing a definitive diagnosis; proctosigmoidoscopy demonstrated bleeding and friability of the mucosa and scraping material from the mucosal surface contained thousands of *E. histolytica* trophozoites. The patient recovered without consequences after metronidazole treatment [16]. It was stated in a previous work that even though no conclusion can be driven by an isolated case report, it is tempting to hypothesize a link between the known histolytic proprieties of *E. histolytica*, the induction of a high inflammatory burden in amoebic infection and its potential induction also of major vessels damage [9]. Additional data that could better inform this hypothesis are strongly needed.

Coronary Aneurysms in Kawasaki Disease Affected by Amoebiasis

Kawasaki disease is an acute febrile illness and systemic vasculitis that predominantly afflicts children of less than 5 years of age; it occurs globally, with an incidence reported in Europe of 5–10 per 100,000 and a male-to-female ratio of 1.5 to 1. It's aetiology, still unknown, is thought to be triggered by an infectious agent [17]. Coronary artery aneurysms were described in paediatric cases of Kawasaki disease, and it was suggested that microorganisms might have a role in the aetiology of the vasculitis that leads to the aneurysm formation in these patients, even though causality couldn't be ascertained [9, 12, 15]. Multiple infectious agents have been previously implicated as triggering agents for Kawasaki Diseases, including viruses, bacteria, rickettsia and candida. In the two cases described by Viswanathan et al., coronary aneurysms occurred with a concomitant diagnosis of amoebic hepatic abscess and Kawasaki disease; a conservative treatment with intravenous immunoglobulins, systemic amoebicidal together with the drainage of the hepatic abscess in one of the two patients was performed. Regression of the coronary lesions was described in these two cases at follow-up [15]. The two cases are summarized in Table 4.1.

Pseudoaneurysms in Amoebic Hepatic Abscess

Vessel involvement in amoebiasis infection was occasionally described in patients with amoebic liver abscess, mostly as pseudoaneurysms [6]. Cases from a previous review of literature are summarized in Table 4.2. Additionally, the pathophysiology of hepatic pseudo-aneurysm development in amoebiasis is described in Fig. 4.2. Independently from their aetiology, hepatic aneurysms are the second most common type of visceral artery aneurysm reported, even though their true actual incidence and natural history are unknown. In the majority of cases, they can be asymptomatic and thus are diagnosed as an occasional finding on imaging performed for other investigations. False aneurysms of the hepatic artery (that account

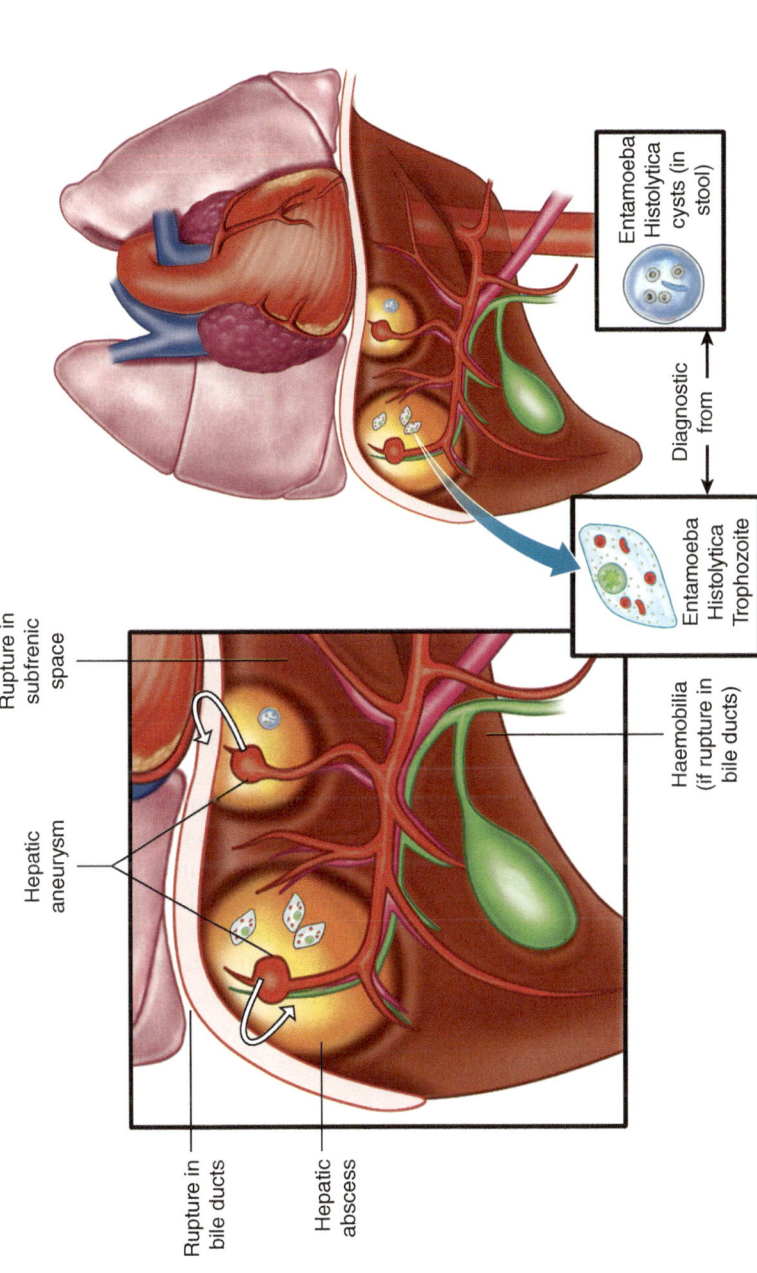

Fig. 4.2 Physiopathology of aneurysm pathology in amoebic liver abscess. Aneurysms may occur due to direct damage from amoebic trophozoite or by damage due to the inflammatory burden. Aneurysms may rupture in various regions including subphrenic space or bile ducts. In this case, haemobilia may occur. Entamoeba histolytic trophozoites may be detected by optical microscopy analysis in samples of abscess; cysts may be seen in stool optical microscopy analysis. The figure was adapted from the original Figure by Valeria Silvestri, from: Silvestri V, Ngasala B. Hepatic aneurysm in patients with amoebic liver abscess. A review of cases in literature. Travel Med Infect Dis. 2022 Mar–Apr; 46:102274. Copyright (2022), with permission from Elsevier

for 25–80% of reported cases) can be secondary to iatrogenic injury or liver trauma, causing gastroenteric bleeding and haemobilia. Rupture of hepatic artery aneurysm was also occasionally described as a complication of this visceral lesion [18].

According to findings from our recent review of cases in literature, hepatic involvement may complicate amoebiasis in patients aged 18–50 years [5]. Aneurysm lesions can thus be diagnosed in patients with amoebiasis at a younger age, if compared to the mean age of patients diagnosed with hepatic aneurysm lesions, which was reported to be 60 years [9, 18] These arterial lesions are also more frequently reported among patients of male gender, with a ratio of 3:2 [9, 18].

As for other lesions of vascular interest affecting patients with NTDs, information related to hepatic artery aneurysm pathology in amoebiasis is only available from small case series, autopsy cases and anecdotal evidence, which have been analysed by our group in a recent review of cases in literature [9]. According to the review results, differently from aneurysms from other aetiologies, which can be diagnosed as occasional findings, all the patients with amoebiasis presenting with hepatic arterial lesions had been assessed because of clinical symptoms. Fever, abdominal pain and anaemia were the most frequently reported features. Haemobilia, hematemesis and melena were found to be the cause of blood loss in four cases [11, 19–21], while occasionally more than one source of bleeding was found [11, 22]. Aneurysm could be diagnosed after treatment of amoebiasis presenting initially with classic intestinal clinical features, as in the case reported by Yanagisawa et al. regarding a 51-year-old patient admitted and treated for perforated appendicitis and peritonitis, in which amoebic trophozoites were found in the colon mucosa. The liver abscess was diagnosed 2 weeks after the emergency intestinal surgery, with the onset of abdominal pain, the appearance of blood in hepatic drainage and cretaceous stool. Rupture of the pseudo-aneurysm into the liver abscess with consequent bleeding from the ampulla of Vater occurred as a complication of intestinal amoebiasis [20].

In addition to aneurysm rupture into the ampulla of Vater, ruptures in other anatomical regions were described. For example, a contained rupture of a right hepatic aneurysm of 10 mm diameter in the sub-phrenic region occurred in a 52-year-old patient with a 2-week history of melena and haemobilia [21]. In a third case, hematemesis and melena were caused by the rupture of a pseudoaneurysm in the seventh branch of the hepatic artery in a 45-year-old patient, after 10 days of history of abdominal pain, fever and hepatomegaly. In this case, complications occurred notwithstanding the 8 days of metronidazole treatment [11]. Bleeding is likely to be the event that brings the patient to medical attention [9].

Diagnostic

The diagnosis of amoebic liver abscess relies on the identification of a space-occupying lesion of the liver and a positive amoebic serology, which is highly sensitive (>94%) and highly specific (>95%). Even though false-negative serological test results can be obtained early in infection (within the first 7–10 days), repeated tests will usually be positive, making this exam extremely useful in the diagnosis of extraintestinal disease [5]. The utility of serological investigations is enhanced in those cases in which direct microscopic assessment for trophozoites and cultural examination for *E. histolytica* in hepatic abscess fluid are negative [23]. We should keep in mind that there could be more than one condition in which an optical microscopic assessment provides a false-negative result. False-negative results for microscopic assessment could occur because of an ongoing metronidazole treatment or because of the user-dependent performance in detecting trophozoites in biological samples that characterize microscopy investigations, which can make this test less sensitive than other diagnostic methods [5]. Mucosal biopsy with direct microscopic research for trophozoites could finally be of help in intestinal manifestations in some cases [20].

Pharmacological Treatment

Anti-amoebic pharmacological treatments exert their action at two different levels: luminal level, where they act only on the intestinal lumen and are so used to treat amoebic non-dysenteric colitis (for example, diiodohydroxyquinoline, paromomycin and diloxanide), and systemic level, which are absorbed in the blood and act in tissues (for example, nitroimidazoles). 5-Nitroimidazoles are a large group active against several protozoan parasites at both the intestinal and tissue levels and are indicated in patients with symptomatic intestinal amoebiasis, hepatic amoebiasis and in asymptomatic cyst carriers. Metronidazole and tinidazole are members of this group [7]. Metronidazole is the preferred pharmacological treatment for patients with amoebiasis, despite its failure to decrease the parasitological state in some cases of resistance (persistence of parasites in stools) and its side effects [7].

In cases with co-occurring vascular lesions, the efficacy of metronidazole to improve and resolve symptoms is not consistent among the reported cases, but intravenous metronidazole every 8 h, together with abscess drainage and intralesional metronidazole cleaning appeared to relieve symptoms due to hepatic amoebic abscess in 72 h and to achieve hepatic aneurysms dimension reduction after 15 days of treatment and its resolution in 2-month follow-up in one case report [23].

Surgical Management

Aneurysms occurring in amebiasis have been reported rarely, and guidelines on its optimal management in this specific setting are lacking [9, 21], thus emphasizing the need to share any additional case that could help to inform the clinical practice of this rarely reported condition of surgical interest.

In the case of hepatic involvement in amoebiasis, we should consider the general guidelines available for hepatic vascular aneurysms. The morbidity and mortality for hepatic artery aneurysm due to rupture reported in literature amount to 30%. Because of the overall low rate of morbidity and mortality after elective repair, the current recommendation is to repair aneurysms >2.0 cm in diameter in low-risk patients and >5.0 cm among high-risk patients, if open repair is planned. In patients with intrahepatic aneurysms, coil embolization of the affected artery has been suggested as the treatment of choice, reserving resection of the involved lobe of the liver to patients with large intrahepatic aneurysms, to avoid the risk of significant necrosis [9, 18].

Endovascular embolization was the most frequently reported procedure to treat pseudo-aneurysms occurring in patients with hepatic amoebiasis, mainly in patients presenting with aneurysm rupture and bleeding [11, 20]. In some cases, embolization could provide resolution of fever, vomiting, jaundice, leucocytosis and normalization of liver function tests, which were persistent notwithstanding hepatic abscess drainage [22]. In all cases included in this chapter, the endovascular embolization of the aneurysm lesion was successful and followed by an uneventful recovery [9]. In those patients treated with embolization, metronidazole treatment alone hadn't been sufficient to solve symptoms related to abscess [21], to stop the development of amoebic abscess [20] nor the development of its vascular complications [11].

While embolization appeared to be successful in endovascularly treated cases, it is of interest that the resolution after abscess drainage and conservative treatment was reported in some cases [21, 23]. The involution of the aneurysm formation in patients with arterial lesions co-occurring with hepatic amoebic abscess could occur because of the liver's capacity to regenerate. In this context, small aneurysm lesions could heal spontaneously after percutaneous drainage because of the removal of necrotic material, bile and blood clots [21]. It is also interesting that a conservative treatment with intravenous immunoglobulins and metronidazole was effective for the conservative management of coronary artery aneurysms occurring in patients with Kawasaki disease, in which the regression of coronary lesions was also documented after treatment [15].

Some parameters were observed that could predict which patient would respond to a conservative approach, including size and location of the aneurysm (with spontaneous resolution more likely for lesions smaller than 2 cm), clinical status and hemodynamic stability of the patient and clinical and radiological response to therapy [9, 21].

Conclusions

Vascular involvement was described in patients with amoebiasis. Notwithstanding the high burden of *E. histolytica* impacting on endemic countries, specifically in low-middle income countries, these complications were described only in sporadic case reports, but the low number of cases could likely be affected by underreporting bias secondary to underdiagnosis and lack of statistical recording in endemic countries. A timely parasitological diagnosis is essential to plan good pharmacological and surgical management in these patients, and it is determinant that clinicians include amoebiasis in the differential diagnosis of patients with vascular presentation, intestinal symptoms and a positive history of potential exposure to *Entamoeba*.

Further studies are needed to better understand this non-communicable vascular complication of a disease of parasitological interest [9].

Acknowledgements This chapter was based on a previous review conducted in our department: *Silvestri V, Ngasala B. Hepatic aneurysm in patients with amoebic liver abscess. A review of cases in literature. Travel Med Infect Dis. 2022 Mar–Apr;46:102274.* A preliminary abstract was presented with title *Hepatic aneurysms in amoebiasis: a review of case reports in literature* during *the BSP Parasites-online meeting, 21–25 June 2021.* Contributors for the abstract presented were, in addition to Valeria Silvestri and Prof Billy Ngasala, Witness M. Bonaventura, from the Kilimanjaro Christian Medical University College, Tanzania; Nyanda C. Justine, Department of Medical Parasitology and Entomology, Catholic University of Health and Allied Sciences, Mwanza, Tanzania; M I Mshana, Parasitology department Muhimbili University of health and Allied sciences and George Ogweno, National Institute for Medical Research, Mwanza, Tanzania.

References

1. Guillén N. Pathogenicity and virulence of Entamoeba histolytica, the agent of amoebiasis. Virulence. 2023;14(1):2158656. https://doi.org/10.1080/21505594.2022.2158656.
2. Speich B, Croll D, Fürst T, Utzinger J, Keiser J. Effect of sanitation and water treatment on intestinal protozoa infection: a systematic review and meta-analysis. Lancet Infect Dis. 2016;16(1):87–99.
3. Le Bailly M, Maicher C, Dufour B. Archaeological occurrences and historical review of the human amoeba, Entamoeba histolytica, over the past 6000 years. Infect Genet Evol. 2016;42:34–40. https://doi.org/10.1016/j.meegid.2016.04.030.
4. Pappas G, Kiriaze IJ, Falagas ME. Insights into infectious disease in the era of Hippocrates. Int J Infect Dis. 2008;12(4):347–50.
5. Stanley SL Jr. Amoebiasis. Lancet. 2003;361(22):1025–34.
6. Silvestri V, Ngasala B. Hepatic aneurysm in patients with amoebic liver abscess. A review of cases in literature. Travel Med Infect Dis. 2022;46:102274. https://doi.org/10.1016/j.tmaid.2022.102274.
7. Carrero JC, Reyes-López M, Serrano-Luna J, Shibayama M, Unzueta J, León-Sicairos N, et al. Intestinal amoebiasis: 160 years of its first detection and still remains as a health problem in developing countries. Int J Med Microbiol. 2020;310(1):151358. https://doi.org/10.1016/j.ijmm.2019.151358.
8. Hotez PJ, Aksoy S, Brindley PJ, Kamhawi S. What constitutes a neglected tropical disease? PLoS Negl Trop Dis. 2020;14(1):1–6.
9. Silvestri V, Ngasala B. Hepatic aneurysm in patients with amoebic liver abscess. A review of cases in literature. Travel Med Infect Dis. 2022;46:102274.
10. Nasrallah J, Akhoundi M, Haouchine D, Marteau A, Mantelet S, Wind P, et al. Updates on the worldwide burden of amoebiasis: a case series and literature review. J Infect Public Health. 2022;15(10):1134–41. https://doi.org/10.1016/j.jiph.2022.08.013.
11. Yadav AK, Gupta S, Hariprasad S, Kumar A, Ghuman SS, Gupta A. Amoebic liver abscess with hepatic artery pseudoaneurysm: successful treatment by interventional radiology. J Clin Exp Hepatol. 2015;5(1):86–8.
12. Viswanathan V. Proceedings of the 24th Paediatric Rheumatology European Society Congress: Part two. Pediatr Rheumatol. 2017;15(S2):65.
13. Fukui A, Nakayama Y, Yoshida T, Murakami K, Kadoba K, Onizawa H, et al. A case of intestinal amoebiasis mimicking intestinal Behçet's disease. Mod Rheumatol Case Rep. 2022;6(2):270–2. https://doi.org/10.1093/mrcr/rxac028.
14. Bettiol A, Alibaz-Oner F, Direskeneli H, Hatemi G, Saadoun D, Seyahi E, et al. Vascular Behçet syndrome: from pathogenesis to treatment. Nat Rev Rheumatol. 2023;19(2):111–26.

15. Viswanathan V, Singh I, Sane S. Amebic liver abscess and Kawasaki disease. Indian Pediatr. 2019;56(6):504–5.
16. Katz S, Romanoff H, Shifrin E. Amoebic dysentery complicating an abdominal aortic aneurys- mectomy. Trans R Soc Trop Med Hyg. 1980;74(6):804–5.
17. Silvestri V. Clinical and surgical features of non-coronary arterial aneurysms in Kawasaki disease: a review of the literature. Prog Pediatr Cardiol. 2021;61:101310. https://doi. org/10.1016/j.ppedcard.2020.101310.
18. Chaer RA, Abularrage CJ, Coleman DM, Eslami MH. The Society for Vascular Surgery clini- cal practice. J Vasc Surg. 2020;72(1):3S–39S.
19. Gopanpallikar A. Hepatic artery pseudoaneurysm associated with amebic liver abscess pre- senting as upper GI hemorrhage. Am J Gastroenterol. 1997;92(8):1391–3.
20. Yanagisawa M, Kaneko M, Aizawa T, Michimata T, Takagi H, Mori M. A case of amebic liver abscess complicated by hemobilia due to rupture of hepatic artery aneurysm. Hepato- Gastroenterology. 2002;49(44):375–8.
21. Priyadarshi RN, Kumar R, Anand U. Case report: spontaneous resolution of intracavitary hepatic artery pseudoaneurysm caused by amebic liver abscess following percutaneous drain- age. Am J Trop Med Hyg. 2019;101(1):157–9.
22. Khan A, Pal KMI, Khan HI. Hepatic artery pseudoaneurysm; a rare complication of amoebic liver abscess. J Pak Med Assoc. 2011;61(8):839–40.
23. Tacconi D, Lapini L, Giorni P, Corradini S, Caremani M. Pseudoaneurysm of the hepatic artery, a rare complication of an amebic liver abscess. J Ultrasound. 2009;12(2):49–52.

Lymphatic Filariasis

5

Contents

Introduction

History of Lymphatic Filariasis: From Manson's Discovery to Ongoing Programmes

In 1876, Sir Patrick Manson returned to Amoy, China, after learning the latest techniques in eye surgery in London. Inspired by an interesting work written by Timothy Lewis in the British Museum library, about the finding of *Filaria sanguinis hominis* in chylous urine and blood of a patient with chyluria, and strong of the fact that he had personally operated previously many patients with elephantiasis who suffered from chyluria, he started to analyse blood samples from patients with elephantiasis.

V. Silvestri et al., *Vascular Damage in Neglected Tropical Diseases*,
https://doi.org/10.1007/978-3-031-53353-2_5

With his compound microscope, he finally observed the presence of abundant sheathed microfilariae [1]. His studies continued, leading to the discovery of the changes in the microfilariae in the alimentary tract and then in the thorax muscles of the mosquito vector of the parasite, a female *Culex fatigans* (*Culex quinquefasciatus*), and, finally, to the discovery of the adult worm of *Wuchereria bancrofti*, in the lymphatic vessels of patients with elephantiasis. The description of the life cycle of filariasis in humans was completed with the observation of nocturnal periodicity, the peak in microfilariae count occurring around midnight, which is sleeping hour for humans, biting hour for vector [1]. Discussed during a meeting of the Linnaean Society of London in 1878, Manson's findings on lymphatic filariasis were described as "*either the work of a genius or more likely the emanation of a drunken Scots doctor in far off China, where they drunk far too much whiskey*" [1].

Even though it officially started in year 2000, the Global Programme for Elimination of Lymphatic Filariasis was built with tools acquired during the entire previous century. After the description by Manson of the lymphatic filariasis life cycle in the 1870s, two potential targets had emerged for the interruption of this disease, respectively: the infected population harbouring the adult helminths together with their micro-filarial stage and the mosquito vectors, which carried the larval infective parasite.

Due to the lack of drugs suitable for infection treatment, the first stage of control programmes focused on vectors [2], but the discovery and the introduction in the clinical practice of diethylcarbamazine in 1947 revolutionized this scenario, and chemotherapy became a predominant strategy for lymphatic filariasis control. While the mechanism of action of this drug is still not totally clear, diethylcarbamazine has a proven microfilaricidal action for both *Wuchereria bancrofti* and *Brugia malayi*, and it is also active against the adult worm stage strategies [2]. For decades after its introduction, approximately 80 countries endemic for lymphatic filariasis used diethylcarbamazine as the principal tool for lymphatic filariasis control, trying various treatment regimens and strategies [2]. The launch of diethylcarbamazine for filariasis treatment was followed in 1980s by the introduction of two other drugs, ivermectin and albendazole, which had already been successfully used in programmes against onchocerciasis [2]. More suitable for African countries that were additionally endemic for *Onchocerca*, the use of ivermectin and albendazole avoided the risk of the intense inflammatory reactions around *Onchocerca* microfilariae that was observed in the skin and the eyes of *Onchocerca* coinfected patients treated with diethylcarbamazine [2].

Diagnostic tools also developed in these early years, to overcome limits of traditional microscopy and serological methods. Microscopic detection of microfilaremia and serologic testing for antibodies were early standard diagnostics for lymphatic filariasis, but the nocturnal periodicity of blood microfilariae and the lack of antibody sensitivity and specificity made them sub-optimal tools for the elimination programme. In response to this, numerous antigen detection diagnostics were developed in the 1980s, and the test based on a monoclonal antibody to parasite antigen AD-12 became the standard for detecting *W. bancrofti* infections in the field [2].

Filariasis causes lymphedema, elephantiasis, hydrocele and acute adeno-lymphangitis, both debilitating and stigmatizing. In the 1990s, the understanding of the pathogenesis of the disease was improved. Ultrasound and lymphoscintigraphic tests allowed to further define the lymphatic involvement that occurs in the infection, visualizing living adults and vessels damage in the form of lymphatic dilatation, compromised function and creation of foci of recurrent bacterial infection, which proved to be critical for the progression of lymphatic damage [2]. It became clear that a clinical management including intensive local hygiene, limb care and prevention of bacterial and fungal infection could provide a dramatic patient improvement thanks to a reduction of acute inflammatory episodes, decreased limb size, reduced stigma and increased quality of life in patients. Additionally, the improvement of surgical approaches for hydrocoele repair increased the efficacy of the overall interventions [2].

In 1997, WHO committed to eliminating lymphatic filariasis as a public health problem at the 50th World Health Assembly, when the burden of lymphatic filariasis was considered to be the second leading cause of chronic disability [3]. In 2020, the Global Programme to Eliminate Lymphatic Filariasis (GPELF) was finally launched to coordinate the comprehensive elimination strategy to reach the elimination of lymphatic filariasis by 2020. The strategy included transmission interruption in endemic communities by use of mass drug administration and the implementation of a morbidity management and disability prevention strategy [3]. Elimination of lymphatic filariasis as a public health problem was first achieved in China in 2007 and South Korea in 2006 [4].

Epidemiology

Lymphatic filariasis is a parasitic disease caused by the filarial nematodes *Wuchereria bancrofti*, *Brugia malayi* and *Brugia timori*, helminths transmitted to humans by several mosquito genera, including *Anopheles*, *Aedes*, *Culex* and *Mansonia* [4, 5]. A long-term infection can affect the lymphatic system, leading to clinical features that include chronic limb lymphedema (that can progress to elephantiasis in severe cases) or to lymphoedema of the scrotum (hydrocele) [4, 5].

After malaria, lymphatic filariasis is the most common vector-transmitted parasitic infection [6]. Its transmission has been documented throughout Africa, Southeast Asia and the Pacific, as well as in focal areas in the Caribbean, South America and the Middle East [4]. According to a model built on a global dataset of 73 georeferenced locations previously known to be endemic for lymphatic filariasis, in the year 2000, a total of 199 million infections were estimated, ranging from approximately 3.1 million in the region of the Americas to approximately 107 million in the South-East Asia region, where 52% of the overall estimated global infections were reported (prevalently in Bangladesh, India, Indonesia and Myanmar). Another 21% of this burden was reported in Africa, (Nigeria, Tanzania, Mozambique and the Democratic Republic of the Congo) [4]. In the African continent, a general decrease in lymphatic filariasis prevalence was reported over the 19-year period during which prevention and control interventions were in place. Globally, the number of individuals infected was reduced by 74%, to an estimated 51 million in 2018. While the global burden of infection is still mostly concentrated in southeast Asia, the highest national prevalence estimates were reported in coastal west Africa, central Africa and Papua New Guinea [4].

The models reflect progress towards elimination, thanks to the programmes that have been designed and implemented [4]. Overall, during the implementation of the GPELF, the prevalence of this disabling disease declined—from approximately 199 million individuals in 2000, to approximately 51 million individuals in 2017; still according to recently published models, not all areas will achieve the original 2020 goal [3]. Up to now, remain 51 countries with ongoing lymphatic filariasis elimination programmes, 15 of which still don't have a full geographic coverage with MDA as of 2018 [4].

While many countries have achieved elimination or are reaching the post-MDA surveillance phase, there is an increasing need to develop strategies to detect transmission in low prevalence settings and determine how to integrate care for patients into the health systems, accounting for changing demographics and mobility overtime [7].

The morbidity management until now was neglected by many elimination programmes in endemic countries, largely slowing down the progress towards a better lifestyle for affected individuals [3]. The earlier studies conducted for the past 20 years mainly focused on lymphatic filariasis transmission control, and very little attention was given to morbidity management and disability prevention, which plays an important role in the transition of lymphedema grades and the frequency of acute attacks. It has been estimated that approximately 15 million people have lymphedema and elephantiasis of the extremities due to filarial parasitic infestation, mainly unilateral but occasionally involving bilateral lower extremity or the upper limbs [8].

Morbidity management practices that include proper limb hygiene, the elevation of the affected limb, pressure garment, proper foot-ware, and treatment for entry lesions are essential to prevent frequency and duration of acute lymphedema attacks, to reduce the progression to higher grades of lymphedema, improve the flexibility, and range of motion of the limbs, reduce chronic inflammatory changes and limb volume [9]. In addition to mass drug administration (MDA) programmes, aiming at the interruption of disease transmission, the management of comorbidity in filariasis lymphedema is an essential component of the global programme to eliminate lymphatic filariasis launched in 2000 by the global alliance to eliminate lymphatic filariasis and include hygiene measures, physiotherapy and surgical hydrocelectomy [5].

New milestones and targets for elimination of lymphatic filariasis as a public health problem have been proposed by WHO, in line with 2030 objectives for Sustainable Development Goals [6].

Clinical Features

The asymptomatic infestation is the most common in lymphatic filariasis, and filariasis may likely be diagnosed occasionally or during screening: two out of three infected people are asymptomatic, even when they have microfilaremia [9, 10]. In patients who do manifest clinical symptoms, lymphatic filariasis can cause severe clinical manifestations, including lymphedema of the limbs or genitals, acute lymphangitis attacks, hydrocele, chyluria, which make lymphatic filariasis to be highly ranked among the disability causing disease. The acute adeno-lymphangitis is clinically characterized by pain that affects people's occupation, income and production, with a global loss of 5.9 million disability-adjusted life years [9]. Long-term infection can cause deterioration of the lymphatic system, characterized by severe swelling of the affected region, including lymphedema of the limb or hydrocele when it involves the scrotum [5]. As the disease progresses to a more severe stage, the legs' volume increases along with the worsening of the oedema, with nodule formation, ulceration and lymphorrhea. Lymphedema is a risk factor for acute bacterial infection, frequently *Streptococcus* spp. in the form of acute dermato-lymph-angio-adenitis. Local pain, embarrassment and limited physical activities are the main distressing aspects of lymphatic filariasis that reduce quality of life and cause socio-psychological negative impact on both patients and their families [8], as observed for many skin-neglected chronic conditions with visible lesions [11]. People who are physically impaired by LF may live for years with disability, stigmatization and mental health co-morbidity [12].

In addition to the most frequent clinically reported presentations of lower limb lymphedema and hydrocele, filariae were detected in cytological smears from various body sites in clinically unsuspected cases of lymphatic filariasis, occasionally associated with malignancy [13]. In the majority of malignant lesions in which filariae were accidentally observed, transient or absent micro-filariaemia was reported in the peripheral blood [13–16]. An intense inflammatory reaction surrounding the parasite was found in histological examination, suggesting that the rich vascular supply of malignant lesions could possibly encourage the concentration of parasites at such sites [10, 13]. Among the types of malignancy in which filariae have been described, we can list haematological malignancies [17–21] including acute lymphoblastic leukaemia [17], chronic myeloblastic leukaemia [19], multiple myeloma [18, 20], solid malignancy in the form of a primary cutaneous diffuse large B-cell lymphoma [21]. In these haematological cases, microfilariae were observed in bone marrow cytology [17] and histology [18, 20] or in peripheral blood [19]. Filariae were also detected in mammary gland [14, 15, 22–25], ovarian malignancies including cysto-adenocarcinoma [26] and cystic teratoma [27]. In males, filarial granuloma can be formed in the tunica testis [28, 29] or in prostatic tissue [30]. Lung and pleural involvement was observed in the form of eosinophilic pneumonia [31, 32] or adenocarcinoma of the lung [13,

20, 22]. Pleural involvement was described as a result of metastatic spread [13, 31, 33]. Finally, microfilariae were detected in metastatic lymph nodes [14, 20, 22, 23, 34] emphasizing the role of cytological screening in metastatic lymph nodes in areas endemic for lymphatic filariasis, even in the absence of clinical symptoms of filariasis [34].

A diagnosis of lymphangiosarcoma was described among the malignant lesions co-occurring with lymphatic filariasis, and is the specific topic of this chapter [35–40],

Diagnosis and Diagnostic Tools

Current guidelines for filaria transmission assessment surveys, to check prevalence after massive drug administration, rely on the detection of circulating filarial antigen in the blood by using antigenic tests such as the filariasis test strip. However, with this method, common filarial antigens can be detected in human blood for years after treatment has cleared microfilariae [41]. A specific diagnosis thus requires demonstration of worms or microfilaria on biopsy or fine needle aspiration cytology [10].

Colour Doppler ultrasound investigations can be additionally useful for the assessment of patients with live intra-lesion microfilariae in many districts, providing the classic ultra-sound diagnostic feature named "filarial dance", generated by the vigorous movement of microfilariae in fluid-filled lesions or dilated lymphatics, which can be detected by the probe [42–44]. Differently from hematic flow, on colour Doppler imaging, filariae provide an irregular non-pulsatile signal [45]. In addition to the ability of localizing the adult worm, ultrasound allows the assessment of the response of the parasite to chemotherapy [46], and it is an essential tool for clinical assessment and research purposes [45]. Many clinical applications have been described for colour Doppler ultrasound in the study of malignant or non-malignant lesions in which lymphatic filariasis can occur, as in mammary gland nodules [47] or lesions of the testis [48].

Pharmacological Treatment

The strategy to interrupt transmission depends on mass drug administration with three anti-parasitic drugs: albendazole, diethylcarbamazine and ivermectin (in different combinations depending on co-endemicity with loaiasis and onchocerciasis and status of MDA programme [11, 49]. Studies have emphasized the importance of adopting triple therapy for the eradication of lymphatic filariasis, with some limitations: specifically, WHO does not recommend the use of triple therapy in countries with endemic *Loa-loa* or *Onchocerca volvulus,* as diethylcarbamazine can cause severe adverse events in people with severe infection with these filaria parasites [49].

Surgery and Lymphatic Filariasis

Among the NTDs prioritized by World Health Organization that are of surgical interest and together with trachoma, lymphatic filariasis is one of the diseases impacting the most on populations DALY in endemic countries, accounting for 2.3 million years lost to disability [50]. From this surgical perspective of morbidity management in NTDs, hydrocele is the most considered manifestation of lymphatic filariasis. Up to 83% of the total economic cost of lymphatic filariasis in India and Africa was considered attributable to this condition involving the scrotum. In 2019, 547,953 hydrocele cases across 56 of 72 endemic countries were reported to the WHO Programme to end lymphatic filariasis; these numbers are likely to be under-estimated because of challenges with data collection in remote areas. Most people with hydroceles require hydrocelectomy for treatment, and continued efforts to treat these patients are essential for both reducing disease burden and for surveillance [50]. Additional feature of surgical interest in patients with lymphatic filariasis, rarely reported, can directly involve the vascular system. Among these, there is lymphangiosarcoma, which is described in detail in the following section.

Overall, the chronic sequelae of surgical interest of NTDs represent a significant driver of morbidity for endemic communities. As stated in the introduction to this book, surgery is recognized as key to enhancing global health to achieve the Sustainable Development Goals, but large gaps still exist in global surgical care, in terms of surgical infrastructure, human resources, financing and education [51]. These gaps in service constitute a barrier to the implementation of morbidity management interventions in low/middle-income countries [52], including those targeting NTD morbidity. Additional factors linked to NTD epidemiology can impair the delivery of effective surgical services in endemic settings. Climate change affects the endemicity scenario of NTDs and can increase the burden of their morbidity management in unprepared regions. The potential disruption of preventive and control interventions in place by unpredictable global events could lead to more surgical cases diagnosed at later and more disabling stage. These considerations emphasize the vulnerability of morbidity management to external events, together with the importance of intensifying and strengthening this specific aspect of current programmes [50].

To fully reach the new roadmap goals for 2021–2030, key actions and programmatic shifts need to be set up to drive progress towards a world free of NTDs by 2030 [53], and these key actions definitely include the strengthening of quality surgical services.

Vascular Damage of Surgical Interest in Lymphatic Filariasis

Lymphangiosarcoma in Lymphatic Filariasis

Lymphangiosarcoma is described as a complication of chronic lymphoedema in rarely reported cases in literature [35–40]. The true incidence of lymphangiosarcoma in chronic filariasis is unknown, and it is likely affected by under-reporting bias in endemic regions [37].

The published case reports in literature were reviewed by our group, by consulting PubMed, EMBASE and Scopus databases using the keywords "filariasis" AND "lymphangiosarcoma" OR "Stewart-Treves syndrome", to carry out a descriptive analysis of anagraphic data, clinical details and surgical management that were available in each report. The retrieved cases are summarized in Table 5.1. Findings showed that the mean age of patients is approximately of 45 years ranging from 19 years to a maximum of 67 years. Lymphangiosarcoma is usually diagnosed in all patients after a long history of chronic lymphatic filariasis, with a mean history of approximately 20 years of chronic condition. The late occurrence of malignancy in patients with a long chronic history of lymphatic filariasis is in line with previous reports on Stewart-Treves Syndrome (lymphangiosarcoma complicating lymphedema secondary to other conditions rather than filariasis) which usually develops in the lower extremity on a history of chronic lymphedema lasting 10–15 years [6]. A recent Chinese monocentric experience by Hao et al. reporting on non-filarial Stewart-Treves syndrome observed a mean duration of lymphedema among patients of 13 years, ranging from 6 months up to 60 years [54].

Before lymphangiosarcoma reaches a definitive diagnosis, the skin lesions can be present from 2 to 24 months, frequently with a concomitant lymphadenopathy. Pain, anaemia secondary to bleeding and an overlapping infection can also be present. The majority of lesions described are ulcerative, characterized frequently by bleeding and foul smell.

Differential diagnosis of lymphangiosarcoma's clinical presentation may be challenging. This specific vascular malignancy, which accounts for 5% of angiosarcoma lesions, should be differentiated from other conditions such as benign vascular proliferation or Kaposi's sarcoma [6]. In some cases, the presence of a benign lymphangiomatosis can be a precursor lesion for the malignant angiosarcoma [38]. This occurred in a case reported by Tambe et al., in which a malignant evolution with recurrent angiosarcoma occurred on a limb's amputation stump, following a first diagnosis of infected capillary haemangioma [6]. In other cases, misdiagnosis can occur, as in the case reported by Muller, in which cutaneous lesions with inguinal lymphadenopathy and fever in a 19-year-old man were erroneously diagnosed as Kaposi sarcoma. The patient was reassessed in another centre after the failure of chemotherapy and radiotherapy [37].

Lymphangiosarcoma is not the only malignancy that has been described in the context of chronic lower limb lymphatic filariasis, but also melanoma [64] and cutaneous B-cell lymphoma [21] have been occasionally described. In order to allow an efficient differential diagnosis, any suspicious lesion should be biopsied [40].

Pathophysiology of Malignancy Co-occurring in Lymphatic Filariasis

The majority of reports have considered the finding of microfilariae in oncological lesions a casualty. But other authors have tried to explain this co-occurrence, defining a list of mechanisms by which it can occur [55]. Among the mechanisms that

Table 5.1 Summary of lymphangiosarcoma in lymphatic filariasis case reports retrieved in literature

N	Author, year	Age	Sex	Diagnosis of LF (years)	Appearance of LAS lesions (months)	Associated conditions	Location of lesion	Clinical presentation	Treatment	Outcome
1	Devi 1977	46	M	25	n.s.	n.s.	Lower limb	Nodular and ulcerating skin lesions (0.5–2 cm); lymphadenopathy	Not offered	EXITUS unknown cause (1 month)
2	Sordillo 1981	40	n.a.	20	n.s.	n.s.	Lower limb	Two large, soft tissue tumour masses	Above the knee amputation and radical lymphadenectomy	ALIVE Lung and peritoneum metastasis (8 years f.u.)
3	Muller 1987	19	M	15	24	Previous chemotherapy and radiotherapy (wrong diagnosis of Kaposi sarcoma)	Leg and dorsal foot	Red nodular tumours; inguinal lymphadenopathy; fever	Hindquarter amputation	ALIVE (24 months-no metastasis)
4	Bhagyalakshmi 2011	38	F	20	2	n.s.	Lateral leg	Enlarging, bleeding ulcerative lesion 12 × 10 cm, lymphadenopathy	Above the knee amputation	ALIVE doing well (6 months f.u.)
5	Krishnamoorthy 2012	67	M	33	12	n.s.	Medial proximal Leg (shin)	Multiple nodules largest ulcerated lobulated (6 × 6 × 2 cm). Muscle invasion	Above the knee amputation	EXITUS Lung metastasis (3 months)

(continued)

Table 5.1 (continued)

N	Author, year	Age	Sex	Diagnosis of LF (years)	Appearance of LAS lesions (months)	Associated conditions	Location of lesion	Clinical presentation	Treatment	Outcome
6	Acharya 2013	36	F	20	4	n.s.	Medial leg	Fungating mass on reddish nodule (10 cm × 7 cm)	Below the knee amputation	ALIVE Free of metastasis on f.u.
7	Agale 2013	50	M	25	3	n.s.	Chronic limb filariasis	Two bleeding nodules of 2–3 cm; inguinal lymphadenopathy	n.s.	n.s.
8	Tambe 2018	64	M	10	4	Previous diagnosis of infected capillary haemangioma Anaemia (bleeding of ulcers)	Antero-lateral leg	Multiple nodular bleeding enlarging lesions with discharge	Above the knee amputation. Palliative chemotherapy on lesion recurrence (paclitaxel)	ALIVE Recurrent lesion on amputation stump. No improvement with paclitaxel. Lost to f.u.
9	Walke 2022	Young age (n.s.)	M	10	Few months	Anaemia (sickle cell)	Anterior leg (shin)	Two ulcero-proliferative lesions (7 × 6 × 3.4 cm); pain Lymphadenopathy	Above knee amputation	ALIVE Disabled (6 months f.u.)

Time since appearance of chronic lymphatic filariasis features is reported (in years), as time since appearance of angiosarcoma lesions (in months). Data on clinical presentation, treatment and outcome (where available) are summarized in columns

M male, *F* female, *n.s.* not specified, *f.u.* follow-up

can likely underlie the finding of filariae in malignancy we can list: the obstruction of vascular and lymphatic vessels; a tumour hyper-vascularity; the inflammation and spread of both tumoral cells and filariae through lymphatics; a likely opportunistic nature of the parasitic disease [14, 30, 33, 56–58] and the production of toxic mediators or the chronic mechanical irritation at the sites of infestation [18].

Obstruction Mechanism

Filaria parasites can circulate in the vascular and lymphatic systems. They may be observed entrapped in tissue fluids or in cytological specimens secondary to a lymphatic obstruction due to scars or tumour compression [14, 56]. Microfilariae circulating in the blood and lymphatics may migrate aberrantly to previously defined "dead-end sites" if there is blockage or damage of the vessels by tumour, inflammation, trauma or stasis [57]. The obstruction of lymphatics by the adult form of the parasite could also lead to peculiar patterns of metastasis of a primary malignancy [30].

Hypervascularity Mechanism

Tumour hypervascularity is a mechanism by which filariae may seed neoplastic tissue. Larvae may be present in the increased lesion's vasculature at the time of cytological sampling, during aspiration: any rupture of vessels during puncture may result in haemorrhage and release of microfilariae [14, 56].

Inflammatory Mechanism or Spread with Atypical Lymphoid Cells

Inflammation, trauma or stasis is another mechanism by which filariae may seed tumours [14, 56].

Opportunistic Nature

Some authors have interestingly suggested the potential opportunistic nature of filarial infection [58]. Some similarities in the immune-modulatory patterns that underline both tumoral and filarial pathology were described. Parasites and tumours have developed strategies of immune-evasion through the expansion of T regulatory cells, the production of inhibitory cytokines or by altering the function of antigen presenting cells with an overall reduction of the activation of T cells. It is known that monocytes and macrophage cells can respond to immunological stimuli according to distinct patterns, and both parasites and tumours alter the balance of monocyte /macrophage sub-populations [13].

Pathophysiology of Lymphangiosarcoma in Lymphatic Filariasis

Differently from other cases in which filariasis co-occurred with malignancy [13–16, 25, 30, 59, 60], in which microfilariae were observed in cytological specimens of different oncological conditions [17, 22], in the cases of lymphangiosarcoma included in our review, malignancy exclusively occurred on chronic lymphedema, and no vital parasite was found in lesions [61]. Instead,

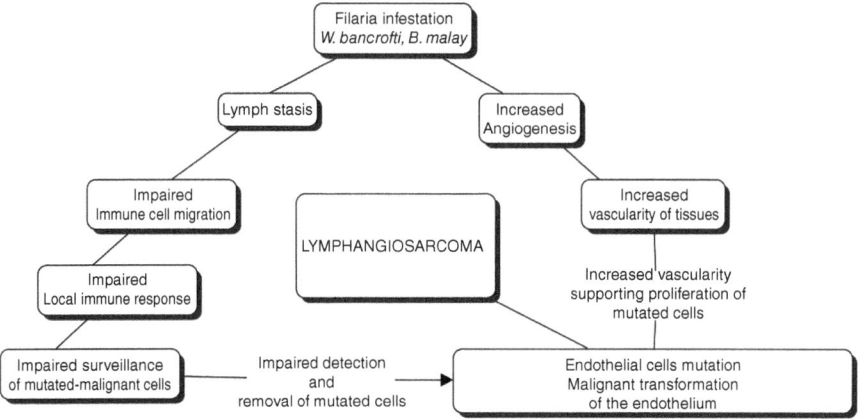

Fig. 5.1 Physiopathology of Lymphangiosarcoma in patients with chronic lymphatic filariasis

granulomatous calcifications of soft tissue attributed to mineralized, degenerated adult filarial worms were described as sign of previous infection [37].

The development of vascular oncogenesis in patients with lymphatic filariasis could thus be secondary mainly to lymph stasis, which impairs immune cell migration, local immune response and angiogenesis [61]. Chronic lymphatic stasis can stimulate angiogenesis and the development of a dense lymphatic and blood vascular network in which malignant transformation of endothelium can eventually occur and develop, whenever a failure of the local mechanisms of immune surveillance for malignant cells occurs [39] (Fig. 5.1).

Surgical Management and Outcome

Major amputation above or below the knee is a frequently performed treatment in patients with lymphangiosarcoma that is diagnosed on chronic lymphatic filariasis. It has been suggested previously that a potential latency of the tumour could justify radical surgery, as major amputation, in the attempt to achieve eradication of local disease [37]. Some of the published cases in literature were actually clear from metastasis on follow-up [40, 62].

Disability due to the demolitive procedure was reported as chronic impairment secondary to the disease [61]. Recurrent lesions on amputation stump have also been described as a late complication of demolitive surgery in these cases [63]. Metastasis notwithstanding demolitive treatment has also been described [40], in one case leading to exitus [39].

Conclusions

As a conclusive remark of this chapter, it is recommended that patients suffering from chronic filarial lymphedema should be monitored for possible development of lymphangiosarcoma with prompt biopsy of suspicious lesions [40]. Further studies are needed that could better assess prevalence and clinical features of this rarely reported co-occurrence of lymphatic filariasis in endemic regions.

Acknowledgements Dr Valeria Silvestri is greatful to Dr Akili Kalinga and to Dr Winfrida John (National Institute of Medical Research-Dar es Salaam), for the opportunity to directly observe the intense clinical and research work related to lymphatic filariasis in Tanzania, and for sharing their professional experience and perspectives.

References

1. To KK, Yuen KY. In memory of Patrick Manson, founding father of tropical medicine and the discovery of vector-borne infections. Emerg Microbes Infect. 2012;1:e31. https://doi.org/10.1038/emi.2012.32.
2. Ottesen EA, Horton J. Setting the stage for a global programme to eliminate lymphatic filariasis: the first 125 years (1875–2000). Int Health. 2021;13:S3–9.
3. Kamgno J, Djeunga HN. Progress towards global elimination of lymphatic filariasis. Lancet Glob Heal. 2020;8(9):e1108–9. https://doi.org/10.1016/S2214-109X(20)30323-5.
4. Deshpande A, Miller-Petrie MK, Johnson KB, Abdoli A, Abrigo MRM, Adekanmbi V, et al. The global distribution of lymphatic filariasis, 2000–18: a geospatial analysis. Lancet Glob Heal. 2020;8(9):e1186–94.
5. Taylor MJ, Hoerauf A, Bockarie M. Lymphatic filariasis and onchocerciasis. Lancet. 2010;2(376):1175–85.
6. An I, Harman M, Ibiloglu I. Topical ciclopirox olamine 1%: revisiting a unique antifungal. Indian Dermatol Online J. 2017;10(4):481–5.
7. Badia-Rius X, Adamou S, Taylor MJ, Kelly-Hope LA. Morbidity hotspot surveillance: a novel approach to detect lymphatic filariasis transmission in non-endemic areas of the Tillabéry region of Niger. Parasite Epidemiol Control. 2023;21:e00300. https://doi.org/10.1016/j.parepi.2023.e00300.
8. Chilgar RM, Khade S, Chen HC, Ciudad P, Yeo MSW, Kiranantawat K, et al. Surgical treatment of advanced lymphatic filariasis of lower extremity combining vascularized lymph node transfer and excisional procedures. Lymphat Res Biol. 2019;17(6):637–46.
9. Mathiarasan L, Das LK, Krishnakumari A. Assessment of the impact of morbidity management and disability prevention for lymphatic filariasis on the disease burden in Villupuram District of Tamil Nadu, India. Indian J Commun Med. 2021;46(4):657–61.
10. Gupta S, Gupta R, Bansal B, Singh S, Gupta KKM. Significance of incidental detection of filariasis on aspiration smears: diagn cytopathol. Diagn Cytopathol. 2009;38(7):517–20.
11. Ending the neglect to attain the Sustainable Development Goals: a strategic framework for integrated control and management of skin-related neglected tropical diseases. Geneva: World Health Organization; 2022. Available at: https://www.who.int/publications/i/item/9789240010352.
12. WHO. Ending the neglect to attain the sustainable development goals: a road map for neglected tropical diseases 2021–2030. WHO; 2020. 196 p.
13. Jha A, Shrestha R, Aryal G, Pant AD, Adhikari RC, Sayami G. Cytological diagnosis of bancroftian filariasis in lesions clinically anticipated as neoplastic. Nepal Med Coll J. 2008;10(2):108–14.
14. Sahoo N, Saha A, Mishra P. Coexistence of microfilaria with metastatic adenocarcinomatous deposit from breast in axillary lymph node cytology: a rare association. J Cytol. 2017;34(1):43–5.
15. Gupta S, Jain S, Sodhani P. Breast carcinoma with co-existent microfilariasis and filarial lymphadenitis diagnosed on cytology. Breast J. 2011;17(1):100–2.
16. Jaiswal S, Chand G, Lal H, Vij MPR. Microfilaria in association with adrenal lymphoma diagnosed on cytology: an extremely rare case. Turk Patoloji Derg. 2013;29(2):143–5.

17. Ashok A, Rakesh K. Acute lymphoblastic leukaemia with microfilaria: a rare coincidence in bone marrow aspirate. Indian J Hematol Blood Transfus. 2011;27(2):111–2.
18. Sharma SCS, Mannan R, Sharma R, Sharma SCS. Microfilaraemia in a case of multiple myeloma: an incidental finding or an association? J Clin Diagnostic Res. 2017;11(12):12–4.
19. Kinger M, Chakrabarti PR, Sharma SKP. Unusual case of bancroftian filariasis co-existing with chronic myeloid leukemia. Ann Trop Med Public Heal. 2014;7(64):6.
20. Kolte S, Mane P. Microfilaria of Wuchereria bancrofti in plasma cell myeloma: a case report. J Vector Borne Dis. 2015;52(4):342–3.
21. Ibrahim S, Jain A, Pai K. A case of false identity: primary cutaneous diffuse large B-cell lymphoma masquerading as Madura foot. Trop Dr. 2021;51(4):617–120.
22. Pantola C, Kala S, Agarwal A, Khan L. Microfilaria in cytological smears at rare sites coexisting with unusual pathology: a series of seven cases. Trop Parasitol. 2012;2(1):61–3.
23. Chakraborty S, Saha M, Pradhan SGBS. Microfilaria infection in metastatic node in a case of breast carcinoma. J Midlife Heal. 2019;10(3):153–5.
24. Atal P, Choudhury MAS. Coexistence of carcinoma of the breast with microfilariasis. Diagn Cytopathol. 2000;22(4):259–60.
25. Thongpiya J, Sa-nguanraksa D, Samarnthai N. Parasitology international filariasis of the breast caused by Brugia pahangi: a concomitant finding with invasive ductal carcinoma. Parasitol Int. 2021;80:102203. https://doi.org/10.1016/j.parint.2020.102203.
26. Vasantham V, Yadav SK, Sarin N, Singh S, Pruthi SK. Incidental detection of microfilaria in cyst fluid of Mucinous cystadenocarcinoma of ovary: a rare case report. Int J Surg Case Rep. 2020;70:56–9.
27. Sane SY, CP. A filarial worm in the wall of a cyst teratoma of the ovary-a case report. J Postgrad Med. 1989;35(4):217–8.
28. Barreto SG, Rodrigues J, Pinto RGW. Filarial granouloma of the testicular tunic mimicking a testicular neoplasm. A case report. J Med Case Rep. 2008;1(2):321.
29. Patne SCU, Das M, Katiyar R. Images in clinical tropical medicine Filarial Orchitis due to Wuchereria bancrofti masquerading as testicular neoplasm. Am J Trop Med Hyg. 2016;95(3):497–8.
30. Malik M, Joseph D, Jonnadula J, Ahmed SF. Case report bilateral testicular metastases and filariasis in prostatic adenocarcinoma. Clin Genitourin Cancer. 2022;15(4):e743–5.
31. Patil PL, Salkar HR, Ghodeswar SS, Gawande JP. Parasites (filaria & strongyloides) in malignant pleural effusion. Indian J Med Sci. 2005;59(10):455–6.
32. Tsanglao WR, Nandan D, Chandelia S, Arya NK, Sharma A. Filarial tropical pulmonary eosinophilia: a condition masquerading asthma, a series of 12 cases. J Asthma. 2019;56(7):791–8.
33. Singh SK, Pujani MP. Microfilaria in malignant pleural effusion: an unusual association. Am J Gastroenterol. 2010;28(4):392–4.
34. Kolte SS, Satarkar RNMP. Microfilaria concomitant with metastatic deposits of adenocarcinoma in lymph node fine needle aspiration cytology: a chance finding. J Cytol. 2010;27(2):2–4.
35. Sordillo EM, Sordillo PP, Hajdu SIGR. Lymphangiosarcoma after filarial infection. J Dermatol Surg Oncol. 1981;7(3)
36. Devi KR, Bahuleyan CK. Lymphangiosarcoma of the lower extermity associated with chronic lymphoedema of filarial origin. Indian J Cancer. 1977;2(14):176–8.
37. Muller R, Hajdu SI, Brennan MF. Lymphangiosarcoma associated with chronic filarial lymphedema. Cancer. 1987;59(1):179–83.
38. Bhagyalakshmi A, Rao GS, Uma P. Cutaneous angiosarcoma in chronic lymphedema: secondary to filariasis. Indian J Surg. 2011;73(5):384–5.
39. Krishnamoorthy N, Viswanathan S, Rekhi B, Jambhekar NA. Lymphangiosarcoma arising after 33 years within a background of chronic filariasis: a case report with review of literature. J Cutan Pathol. 2012;39(1):52–5.
40. Agale SV, Khan WAZA, Chawlani K. Chronic lymphedema of filarial origin: a very rare etiology of cutaneous lymphangiosarcoma. Indian J Dermatol. 2013;58(1):71–3.
41. Greene SE, Fischer K, Choi YJ, Curtis KC, Budge PJ, Mitreva M, King CL, Fischer PUWG. Characterization of a novel microfilarial antigen for diagnosis of Wuchereria bancrofti infections. PLoS Negl Trop Dis. 2022;16(5):1–16.

42. Patil JA, Patil ADRS. Filarial " dance " in breast mass. AJR Am J Roentgenol. 2003;181(4):1157–8.
43. Tai Y, Chiu N, Chi H, Bachmann TT, Huang F, Lin C. Woman with swelling of the left breast. Ann Emerg Med. 2017;70(5):621647.
44. Le Dault E. Incidental mammary calcifications in a Cameroonian migrant: a diagnostic challenge. Travel Med Infect Dis. 2019;28:115.
45. Mand S, Marfo-debrekyei Y, Dittrich M, Fischer K, Adjei O, Hoerauf A. Animated documentation of the filaria dance sign (FDS) in bancroftian filariasis. Filaria J. 2003;2(1):3.
46. Suresh S, Kumaraswami V, Suresh I, Rajesh K, Suguna G, Vijayasekaran V, et al. Ultrasonographic diagnosis of subclinical filariasis. J Ultrasound Med. 1997:45–9.
47. Surendrababu NRS, Thomas E, Rajinikanth J, Edin M, Keshava SN. Breast filariasis: real-time sonographic imaging of the filarial dance. J Clin Ultrasound. 2007;36(9):567–9.
48. Faris R, Hussain O, Setouhy MEL, Ramzy RMR, Weil GJ. Bancroftian filariasis in Egypt: visualization of adult worms and subclinical lymphatic pathology by scrotal ultrasound. Am J Trop Med Hyg. 1999;59(6):864–7.
49. Abuelazm MT, Abdelazeem B, Badr H, Gamal M, Ashraf M, Abd-elsalam S. Efficacy and safety of triple therapy versus dual therapy for lymphatic filariasis: a systematic review and meta-analysis. Trop Med Int Heal. 2022;27(3):226–35.
50. Shirley H, Grifferty G, Yates EF, Raykar N, Wamai R, McClain CD. The connection between climate change, surgical care and neglected tropical diseases. Ann Glob Heal. 2022;88(1):1–6.
51. Alayande BT, Hughes Z, Fitzgerald TN, Riviello R, Bekele A, Rice HE. With equity in mind: evaluating an interactive hybrid global surgery course for cross-site interdisciplinary learners. PLOS Glob Public Heal. 2023;3(5):e0001778. https://doi.org/10.1371/journal.pgph.0001778.
52. Albelbeisi AH, Albelbeisi A, El Bilbeisi AH, Taleb M, Takian A, Akbari-Sari A. Public sector capacity to prevent and control of noncommunicable diseases in twelve low- and middle-income countries based on WHO-PEN standards: a systematic review. Heal Serv Insights. 2021:14.
53. WHO. Neglected tropical diseases. 2023. https://www.who.int/news-room/questions-and-answers/item/neglected-tropical-diseases.
54. Hao K, Sun Y, Zhu Y, Xin J, Zhang L, Li B, et al. A retrospective analysis of Stewart-Treves syndrome in the context of chronic lymphedema. An Bras Dermatol. 2023;98(3):287–95. https://doi.org/10.1016/j.abd.2022.04.011.
55. Babu P, Akabas L, Tariq S, Huda N, Bennuru S, Sabzevari H, et al. Similarities and differences between helminth parasites and cancer cell lines in shaping human monocytes: insights into parallel mechanisms of immune evasion. PLoS Negl Trop Dis. 2018;12(4):1–19.
56. Ahluwalia C. Incidental detection of microfilariae in aspirates from Ewing's sarcoma of bone. Diagn Cytopathol. 2003;29(1):31–2.
57. Aron M, Kapila K, Verma K. Microfilariae of Wuchereria bancrofti in cyst fluid of tumors of the brain a report of three cases. Diagn Cytopathol. 2001;26(3)
58. Mohan S, Andley M, Talwar N, Ravi B, Kumar A. An unusual association with carcinoma pancreas: a case report. Cythopathology. 2005;16(4):215–6.
59. Silvestri V, Sciences A, Mushi V, Sciences A, Mshana M, Sciences A, et al. Filariasis and malignancy: analysis of an association through a narrative review of literature. Tanzan J Health Res. 2022;23:82.
60. Sane SY, Patel CV. A filarial worm in the wall of a cystic teratoma of the ovary—(a case report). J Postgrad Med. 1989;35(4):21–2.
61. Walke VA, Datar S, Kowe B, Chaurasia JK. Unusual coexistence of Stewart-Treves syndrome and sickle cell anaemia: a case of dual pathology. BMJ Case Rep. 2022;15(7):1–4.
62. Acharya AS, Sulhyan KR, Ramteke RV, Kunghadkar VY. Cutaneous lymphangiosarcoma following chronic lymphedema of filarial origin. Indian J Dermatol. 2013;58(1):68–70.
63. Tambe SA, Nayak CS. Metastatic angiosarcoma of lower extremity. Indian Dermatol Online J. 2018;9:177–81.
64. Rekha A, Ravi A, Venu N, Shivanraj A. Malignant melanoma and filariasis: a coexistence or an association? Int J Low Extrem Wounds. 2005;4(1):60–4.

Tungiasis

6

Contents

Introduction

Epidemiology

Tungiasis is a dermatological parasitic disease caused by two of the 13 known species of female sand flea (*Tunga penetrans and Tunga trimammillata*), which affects humans and other mammals [1]. *Tunga* spp. is the smallest known flea, measuring approximately 1 mm in length [2]; together with scabies, the disease is included in the list of NTDs under the definition of "other ectoparasites" [3].

The disease was imported in Africa in 1872 through a British ship arriving at the Angolan port of Ambriz and spreading across the continent through the caravan traffic. The condition rapidly became a threat to the unaware population. Nutritional conditions also worsened the impact of the disease, defined by Meyer as *"the most fearful calamity that has ever afflicted the East African peoples"* which lead to the loss of lives because of complications of untreated lesions such as infection and gangrene [4].

© The Author(s), under exclusive license to Springer Nature
Switzerland AG 2024
V. Silvestri et al., *Vascular Damage in Neglected Tropical Diseases*,
https://doi.org/10.1007/978-3-031-53353-2_6

T. penetrans is now endemic in tropical and subtropical regions of the Caribbean, South America and sub-Saharan Africa [3], where the disease occurs focally, predominantly in urban slum areas, rural settings, fishing villages and indigenous communities [5]. It is also an emerging pathology among travellers from non-endemic areas; walking barefoot on dry and sandy soils or beaches and visiting local communities in endemic settings without insecticide prophylaxis are risk factors for the infestation in travellers [1, 6]. Climate change can lead to seasonal variation in *T. penetrans*, changing the transmission dynamics and increasing the severity of outbreaks due to prolonged and severe dry seasons in endemic areas. Additionally, the infestation is favored by the increasing contact of populations with sylvatic animals, which are important reservoirs for *Tunga* spp. [5].

In endemic settings, the larvae and pupae develop in dry shaded soils, frequently inside the bedrooms of houses with an unsealed earthen floor where most transmission occurs. Even though, according to data from WHO, over one billion people live in areas suitable for tungiasis transmission, because of the lack of routine surveillance at the country level, the actual disease burden is not known [3], and there is currently no globally accepted roadmap for its control [7]. Estimates from Latin America reported that 450 million people are currently living in suitable areas, 347 million in urban and 103 million in rural areas in the continent [5].

In endemic communities, children aged 5–14 years and adults older than 60 years are affected the most, with a prevalence of up to 85% among these groups compared with 50% in the general population. [8]. Recent data from the North-eastern Tanzania observed an overall prevalence of tungiasis infestation among school-age children of 21.2%, recognizing the ecto-parasitosis as a public health problem in the area, with the potential to cause severe disease and deformities in the vulnerable population [9]. A higher prevalence was reported from other African settings, explained by the seasonality of the infestation, affected by the level of dust (that composes *Tunga spp*'s habitat) in the environment. The prevalence of Tungiasis from other Tanzanian settings was reported to range from 39% to 97% [10–12]. Data from Ethiopia showed a prevalence ranging from 23.9% to 52.3% [13], while in Uganda, it was 22.5% [14], and in Nigeria (45%) [15]. Data from Kenya show that in 2014, ten million people were at risk of acquiring Tungiasis, with 1.4 million being infected (4% of the overall population) and 265 deaths that occurred, possibly because of complications such as septicaemia and tetanus [8].

Physiopathology and Clinical Presentation

Tunga penetrans is classified among the ectoparasites. The adult female penetrates the epidermis of the host within 6-8 h. After penetration, the abdominal segment of the ecto-parasite protrudes from the skin surface, where it becomes visible as an enlarging dot. In this site, the parasite eliminates faeces and lays eggs (100–200/week) and accomplishes vital functions such as breathing and copulation [16] while feeding on dermal layers [1]. Once fertilized, the flea undergoes abdominal hypertrophy and grows up to 2000-fold within 1 week. A complete life cycle lasts 4 weeks when the involute parasite is detached through skin exfoliation [16].

The clinical presentation of the ecto-parasitosis includes the appearance of a yellow papule (<3–8 mm) with a dark central dot that corresponds to the enlarged abdomen of a pregnant female. On magnified examination, eliminated eggs are visible in the surrounding skin [16]. Signs and symptoms include itching, skin desquamation, black dots, fissures, digits and nail deformation, constant pain and difficulty walking [9]. Pathophysiology of Tunga spp. infestation is described in Fig. 6.1.

Tungiasis infestation entails chronic sequelae, potentially leading to discomfort, foot deformity, foot mutilation and reduced mobility. Also, in children, it affects school attendance, contributing to poor performance and to dropout rates [9, 15, 17]. In the adult population, severe complications secondary to infection have been described in patients with comorbidities that can impair tissue repair, such as diabetes, potentially leading to death [9, 18].

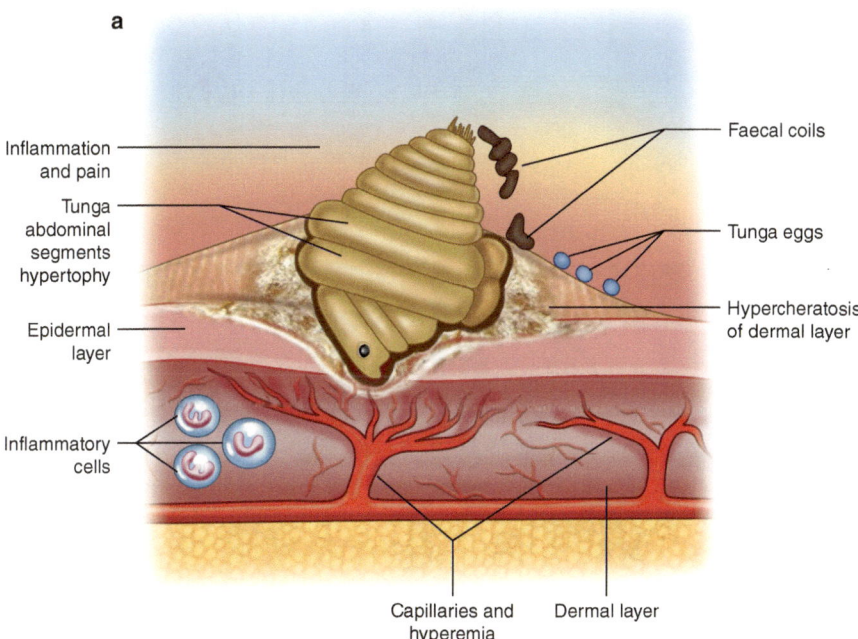

Fig. 6.1 Pathophysiology of Tunga spp. infestation. (**a**) Pictorial view of Tunga penetrans invading epidermis, with hypertrophic changes in abdominal segments. The oviposition and excretion of faeces continues until the parasite's death. Around the parasite, the epidermal layer shows hypertrophic and hyperkeratotic changes. Hyperaemia and inflammatory changes occur in the dermal layer, where T. penetrans acquires nutrients. (**b**) The five stages of Fortaleza classification: (1) invasion by the parasite; (2) complete penetration of epidermis and faecal excretion; (3) hyperkeratotic changes of epidermis and hypertrophic changes of abdominal segments; (4) lesion involution after parasite's death; (5) residual skin abrasion. Complications with infection and necrosis are summarized in the last square. (C) Photographs of lesions at different stages of infection, indicated by a number. Adapted from the original Figure available from: Mtunguja M, Mushi V, Silvestri V, Palilo H, John W, Yangaza YE, Tarimo D. Tungiasis infection among primary school children in Northeastern Tanzania: prevalence, intensity, clinical aspects and associated factors. IJID Reg. 2023 Mar 5;7:116–123

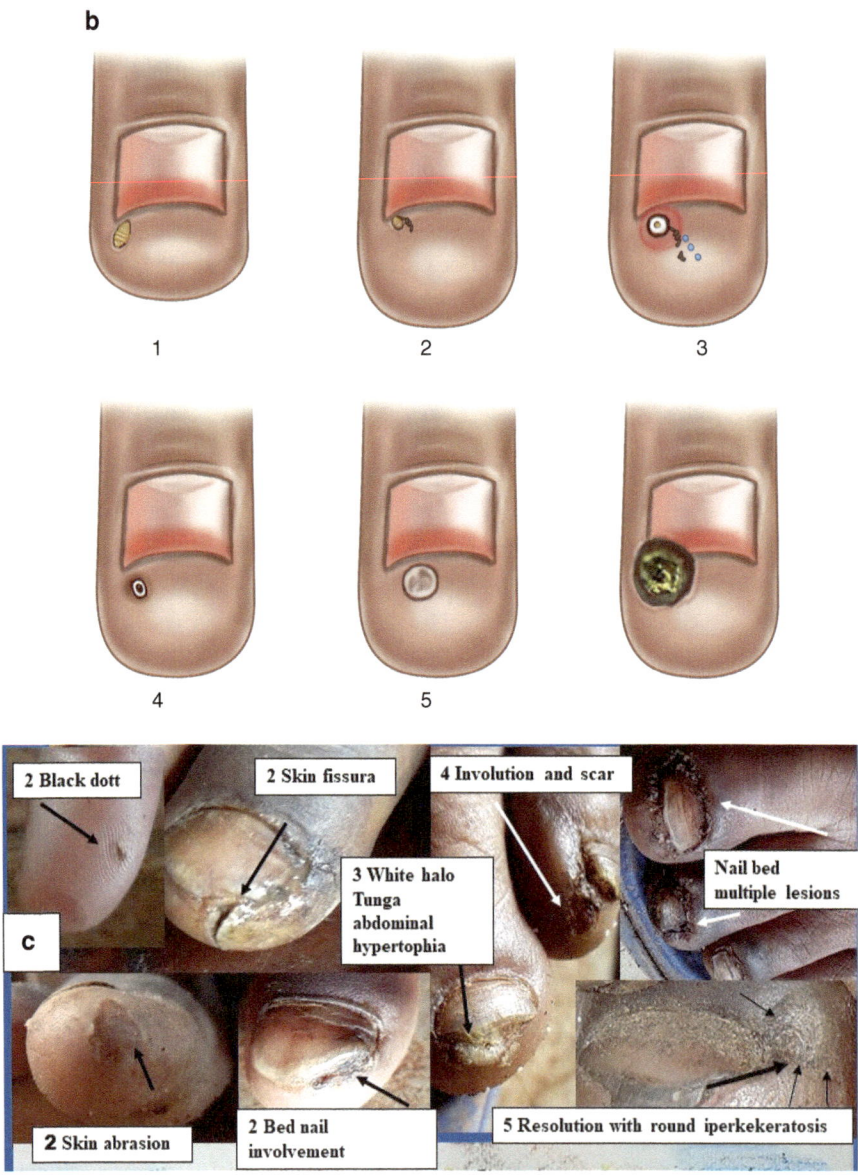

Fig. 6.1 (continued)

Treatment

As occurs in other NTDs with skin manifestations, this condition requires individual case management, which faces the barrier of scarce interest by donors and financial restraints. Differently from diseases mainly managed through mass drug administration (MDA), individual case management is essential for those patients who are already symptomatic, to address the long-term consequences of the disease [19].

A common treatment practised in endemic areas, as reported by WHO, is the surgical extraction of embedded sand fleas using sterile instruments by an experienced health worker at the health facility, followed by topical treatment. Self-extraction using non-sterile instruments in a non-sterile environment is not uncommon, leading to inflammation and bacterial superinfection such as cellulitis and tetanus or transmission of blood-borne infections [2, 9], post-streptococcal glomerulonephritis and sepsis [20].

Vascular Damage in Patients with Tungiasis

Tungiasis can be complicated by the inflammatory burden at the infection site and by overlapping infections [9, 18]. Additionally, iatrogenic inflammation or infection can occur as a result of the diagnostic procedures or of the treatment attempt. The diagnostic incision required for many differential diagnoses in patients with tungiasis, (including warts, granulomas, tropical ulcers, scabies, tick bites, secondary pyoderma, abscesses or malignant melanoma) can result in secondary cellulitis, erysipelas, tetanus or septicaemia, and can alter, by external manipulation, the clinical presentation of tungiasis [21]. Because of the local inflammation at the embedding point in the skin or secondary to the iatrogenic damage during diagnostic or to therapeutic incision, the infection may require, in extreme cases, the amputation of the affected site, more frequently digits. Occasionally other parts of the body may be affected and require demolitive treatment, such as the tongue, in a rare case described by Sentogo et al. in which the patient acquired tungiasis when sleeping on the floor [22].

Amputation may thus occur in patients with no other predisposing factor for it rather than the sequelae of the infestation or the iatrogenic damage manifesting during the treatment attempt. However, in patients with underlying vascular impairment, *Tunga* infestation may represent a significant threat to the affected limb. It is the case of those patients with diabetes complicated by vasculopathy [18]. The pathophysiology mechanisms that can lead to critical ischemia in patients with tungiasis are summarized in Fig. 6.2.

Diabetic foot ulcer complicates chronic diabetic ischemia in 15%–34% of cases. Approximately 50% of diabetic ulcers become infected, and 20% of moderate or severe diabetic foot infections lead to amputation, making diabetic foot among the first causes of major amputation worldwide [23]. Diabetic patients are at risk of developing foot ulcers as a result of many factors, including hyperglycaemia, trauma, underlying diabetic peripheral neuropathy and peripheral arterial disease [18].

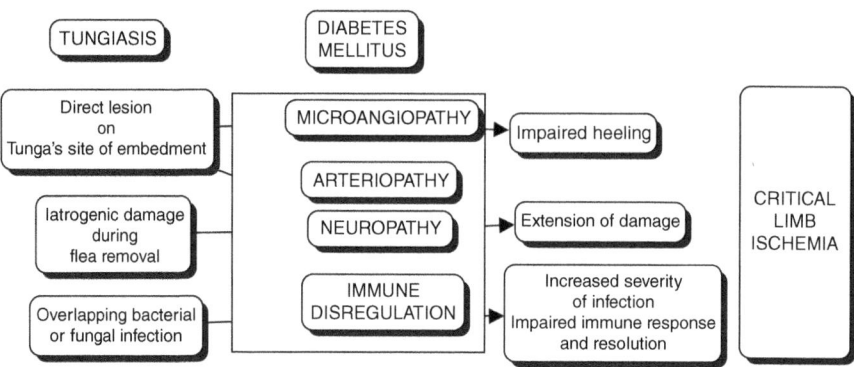

Fig. 6.2 Pathophysiology of vascular damage in Tungiasis. The damage occurring at the site of the ectoparasite embedment, together with iatrogenic lesions or overlapping infection, can occur in patients with complications due to diabetes mellitus (microangiopathy, arteriopathy, neuropathy and impaired immune response to infections). In these patients, the complications occurring on the skin lesion can lead to critical limb ischaemia through impaired healing of extension of damage and increased severity of overlapping infections

To understand the potential threat of tungiasis in low- and middle-income countries in those cases where the parasitic infection overlaps with other diseases that cause vascular disorders, we should first consider the specific epidemiology and associated challenges of diabetes in the regions endemic for NTDs. Data related to the prevalence of clinical manifestations in diabetes mellitus type 2 in Africa show that peripheral vascular disease is observed in 4–28% of cases, that neuropathy underlies diabetic foot more often than peripheral vascular disease and the prevalence of foot ulceration ranges from 4% to 19% [23]. Lower extremity amputation occurs in 1.5–7% of cases [8]. Still, a major concern for low- and middle-income countries is that administrative data are often not used to estimate diabetes-related complication rates due to a lack of data availability and fruition [24], and the above-reported prevalence cound be underestimated.

In diabetes with peripheral neuropathy and vascular impairment, *T.penetrans* infection or the trauma following its extraction may predispose to rapidly progressing ulcer due to healing impairment and can increase the risk of an unfavourable outcome due to sepsis and death [18]. Because of the lack of reliable stats on diabetic burden among those populations also endemic for NTD [24], as observed earlier, this co-occurrence of diabetic complications and *Tunga* coinfection is likely to go underdiagnosed and to be under-reported in endemic settings.

Worsening of Critical Limb Ischemia in Patients with Tungiasis

One isolated but interesting case of worsening of chronic limb ischaemia after *Tunga* infestation was reported by Ebrahim et al. in Dar es Salaam. A 50-year-old woman presented with a 2-week history of a progressing ulcer on her right foot following a cutaneous infestation by a sand flea, *T. penetrans* [18].

The patient, diagnosed with type 2 diabetes mellitus 5 years previously, was not on regular medication for her metabolic condition. After noticing an asymptomatic white "nodular" lesion at the tip of the second toe, and another on the first metatarsal-phalangeal joint, she removed the flea with a non-sterile pin. An abscess developed after pin removal around the wounds, with pain and swelling of the foot, followed within 2 weeks by ulceration extended to the anteromedial aspect of the right foot. Fever, generalized malaise and episodes of fatigue were present. Doppler studies showed a bilateral impairment in peripheral arterial function, leading to a diagnosis of neuro-ischaemic diabetic foot ulcer secondary to *T. penetrans*. Even though symptoms and signs of infection subsided 3 days later, with the achievement of glucose control, the ulcer increased in size, and the ischemic status of the limb led to toe gangrene. After refusing treatment and being discharged on oral antibiotics, the patient was readmitted with sepsis 1 week later and died after 24 h in the intensive care unit [18].

This unique case highlights the many challenges in managing complications of the co-occurrence of this parasitic disease in diabetic populations in NTD endemic settings. Sub-Saharan African countries will likely experience the worldwide fastest increase in the number of people living with type 2 diabetes in the next two decades, but early prevention and control of this metabolic disease are still not sufficiently addressed. The proportion of undiagnosed diabetes in Africa is double the one reported in developed countries (66.7% vs. 37%), contributing to the burden of morbidity and mortality for this metabolic condition at an early age in Africa and to the progress to disabling and life-threatening complications [25], including the one described in this chapter.

The case reported by Ibrahim had been diagnosed 5 years previously but had stopped treatment and incurred in severe metabolic impairment and vascular complications. Additionally, she increased the risk of diabetic complication by self-managing the lesion with non-sterile tools and self-assessment of the ulcer until the chronic limb ischemia evolved into critical limb ischaemia with gangrene, finally threatening her life [18]. This case emphasizes how the overlapping of neglect for both metabolic diseases and the ectoparasitosis can be detrimental in endemic settings and calls to urgently address this issue with further population-based studies, inquiring on the prevalence, features and outcome of the co-occurrence of these diseases.

Conclusions

Tungiasis is a neglected yet significantly prevalent condition in endemic tropical and subtropical regions of the Caribbean, South America and sub-Saharan Africa. Its potential interaction with non-communicable diseases like diabetes and the increasing burden of this metabolic condition in low- and middle-income countries call for studies that will better define the prevalence and clinical features of the co-occuring condition and will inquire on the prevalence of diabetes type 2 complications in terms of ulcers, bacterial infection or worsening of chronic limb ischaemia in diabetic patients that are also affected by tungiasis. Findings will eventually guide preventive interventions towards a specific parasitological potential vascular threat during times of general rise of non-communicable diseases in endemic settings.

References

1. Palicelli A, Boldorini R, Campisi P, Disanto MG, Gatti L, Portigliotti L, et al. Tungiasis in Italy: an imported case of Tunga penetrans and review of the literature. Pathol Res Pract. 2016;212(5):475–83. https://doi.org/10.1016/j.prp.2016.02.003.
2. Cagnon GV, Carvalho Dos Santos D, Miot HA. Tungiasis. JAMA Dermatol. 2019;155(10):1181.
3. WHO. Tungiasis. 2023. Available from: https://www.who.int/news-room/fact-sheets/detail/tungiasis.
4. Kjekshus H. Ecology control and economic development in East African history: case of Tanganyika. 2nd ed. Ohio: Ohio University Press; 1996.
5. Deka MA, Heukelbach J. Distribution of tungiasis in latin America: identification of areas for potential disease transmission using an ecological niche model. Lancet Reg Health Am. 2022;5 https://doi.org/10.1016/j.lana.2021.100080.
6. Shepard Z, Rios M, Solis J, Wand T, Henao-Martínez AF, Franco-Paredes C, et al. Common dermatologic conditions in returning travelers. Curr Trop Med Rep. 2021;8(2):104–11.
7. Elson L, Wright K, Swift J, Feldmeier H. Control of tungiasis in absence of a roadmap: grassroots and global approaches. Trop Med Infect Dis. 2017;2(3):1–13.
8. Motala AA. Type 2 diabetes mellitus in sub-Saharan Africa: challenges and opportunities. Nat Rev Endocrinol. 2022;18(4):219–29.
9. Mtunguja M, Mushi V, Silvestri V, Palilo H, John W, Yangaza YE, et al. Tungiasis infection among primary school children in Northeastern Tanzania: prevalence, intensity, clinical aspects, and its associated factors. IJID Reg. 2023;7:116–23.
10. Mazigo HD, Bahemana E, Konje ET, Dyegura O, Mnyone LL, Kweka EJ, et al. Jigger flea infestation (tungiasis) in rural western Tanzania: high prevalence and severe morbidity. Trans R Soc Trop Med Hyg. 2012;106(4):259–63.
11. Dassoni F, Polloni I, Margwe SB, Veraldi S. Tungiasis in Northern Tanzania: a clinical report from Qameyu village, Babati District, Manyara Region. 2014.
12. Mazigo HD, Behamana E, Zinga M, Heukelbach J. Tungiasis infestation in Tanzania, vol. 4. J Infect Dev Ctries; 2010. p. 187–9.
13. Jorga SD, Dessie YL, Kedir MR, Donacho DO. Prevalence of tungiasis and its risk factors of among children of Mettu woreda, Southwest Ethiopia, 2020. PLoS One. 2022;17(1):e0262168.
14. Wafula ST, Ssemugabo C, Namuhani N, Musoke D, Ssempebwa J, Halage AA. Prevalence and risk factors associated with tungiasis in Mayuge district, Eastern Uganda. Pan Afr Med J. 2016;24:77.
15. Ugbomoiko US, Ofoezie IE, Heukelbach J. Tungiasis: high prevalence, parasite load, and morbidity in a rural community in Lagos State, Nigeria. Int J Dermatol. 2007;46(5):475–81.
16. Krüger GM, Takita LC, Loro LS, Hans FG. Disseminated tungiasis. An Bras Dermatol. 2017;92(5):727–8.
17. Enwemiwe VN, Ojianwuna CC, Anyaele OO. Intensity and clinical morbidities of tungiasis in an impoverished south-west Nigerian community. Parasite Epidemiol Control. 2021;14:e00215.
18. Ebrahim AA, Mpango EP, Temba JA, Abbas ZG, Mashili FL. Tunga penetrans causing a rapidly progressing foot ulcer in a patient with uncontrolled type 2 diabetes mellitus. Oxford Med Case Rep. 2022;2(3):85–8.

19. World Health Organization. Ending the neglect to attain the sustainable development goals: a strategic framework for integrated control and management of skin-related neglected tropical diseases 2021–2030. WHO (World Health Organization). 2022:1–61. http://apps.who.int/bookorders

20. Abrha S, Heukelbach J, Peterson GM, Christenson JK, Carroll S, Kosari S, et al. Clinical interventions for tungiasis (sand flea disease): a systematic review. Lancet Infect Dis. 2021;21(8):e234–45.

21. Beg MA, Saleem T, Zubari A, Mehraj V, Yakoob N, Zafar H, et al. Tungiasis: consequences of delayed presentation/diagnosis. Int J Infect Dis. 2008;12(2):218–9.

22. Sentongo E, Wabinga H. Tungiasis presenting as a soft tissue oral lesion. BMC Oral Health. 2014;14(1):1–4.

23. Ruhembe C, Mosha TCE, Nyaruhucha C. Prevalence and awareness of type 2 diabetes mellitus among adult population in Mwanza city, Tanzania city, Tanzania. Tanzan J Heal Res. 2014;16(2):89–97.

24. Ali MK, Pearson-Stuttard J, Selvin E, Gregg EW. Interpreting global trends in type 2 diabetes complications and mortality. Diabetologia. 2022;65(1):3–13.

25. Wolde HF, Derso T, Biks GA, Yitayal M, Ayele TA, Gelaye KA, et al. High hidden burden of diabetes mellitus among adults aged 18 years and above in urban Northwest Ethiopia. J Diabetes Res 2020;2020.

Contents

Introduction

Epidemiology of Snakebites

Snake envenomation is an issue of public health concern, involving all continents except for Antarctica [1]. Currently, about 4000 species of venomous snakes are recognized, including 389 *Elapidae*, such as cobras, mambas, coral snakes, kraits and sea snakes, and 374 *Viperidae*, such as vipers, adders, rattlesnakes and other pit vipers; these two families are responsible of most snakebite envenoming worldwide [2]. Among these, WHO identified 113 most important medical species in different countries and another 157 species that deserve prioritization for antivenom coverage [2].

The medical interest for snakes and envenomation is antique, and it is documented in ancient Egyptian papiry. The Brooklyn Papyrus, housed in the Brooklyn Museum, believed to be a copy dating to the Late period (664–332 BCE) based on an earlier original, contained guidelines for the priests of the goddess Serqet, who were called upon to treat those who had been bitten by snakes. It contains a description of various snakes, describes the effects of their bites and the prognosis for the bite victims [3]. According to Galen (De theriaca ad Pisonem: 237), in ancient Egypt *"human and prompt executions' were obtained in Alexandria with the intervention of cobras"*, sentence that proves the insistent use of venoms in that period [4]. The last member of Ptolemaic Dynasty, queen Cleopatra VII, also manifested the great inclination of Ptolemies towards medicine and science. The queen committed suicide in August 30 BC, and according to Strabo, *"she too put herself to death secretly, while in prison, by the bit of an asp or by applying a poisonous ointment"* [4].

Worldwide, the estimated number of annual deaths due to snake envenomation ranges from 80,000 to 130,000, with the lowest occurrence reported in Europe [1] and the highest occurrences in Asia and Africa, where mortality is also higher due to inequality in access to treatment [1]. Still, global epidemiological data are likely to underestimate the burden of this public health threat in terms of incidence, morbidity and prevalence of chronic sequelae. The neglect faced by this condition as a public health problem [2], the lack of coordinated data collection and the fact that not all the clinical cases arrive for medical attention can suggest that the incidence of snakebite envenomation is likely to be underestimated and that data describing the related morbidity and mortality due to this condition are likely to be incomplete [5]. Examples from countries of sub-Saharan Africa, such as the Democratic Republic of Congo, which have a high population density and a considerable presence of medically important snakes, can't but highlight the deficiencies of currently accepted estimates of global snakebite mortality [2]. Well-conducted epidemiological studies from other settings reported that only in Asia the total snakebite mortality exceed 66,000, making unrealistic the global estimations [2].

Children are at increased risk of death after snakebite envenomation: younger age is a risk factor likely due to the lower body mass of children that determines a smaller volume of distribution of venom [5]. Snakebites and death from envenomation are most frequent in rural, low-income regions, where barriers to rapid health care access and antivenom administration are the norm, and intensive supportive care can be unavailable [1]. Previous studies have emphasized that residing in rural areas and walking for more than 1 km after envenoming are factors associated with increased mortality after envenoming. Challenges and delays in the access of patients to health services, poor availability of antivenoms and other therapeutic devices, the shortage of medical and nursing personnel and non-adherence to therapeutic protocols for managing snakebite envenoming and its complications may also contribute to the increased morbidity and mortality in endemic areas [5].

Among patients who survive, delayed or inadequate care can lead to permanent disabilities such as amputations or blindness [1].

WHO added snakebites to the list of NTD in 2017, an action that was followed in 2018 by the 71st World Health Assembly resolution on snakebite, and in 2019, by the launch of the associated WHO strategy to halve snakebites' burden by 2030 [5]. Furthermore, the WHO strategy focuses on the chronic aspects of snakebite care, towards the decrease of not only mortality but also morbidity by 50% by 2030 [6] through preventive efforts, improved treatments and enhanced access to care [1]. In this perspective, it is important to strengthen the healthcare systems, increasing the availability of antivenoms and the necessary professional expertise in the centres treating the condition. In addition, it is important to encourage studies focusing on specific aspects of this neglected tropical condition [6] and to standardize the outcome measures in reports that could guide future investigationsneeded to fulfil this aim [7].

The acceptance of snakebite envenoming within the NTD community is still considered a challenge, due to the fact that it *"opened the NTD categories to non-infectious diseases"* [5]. Vascular lesions occurring as a result of snakebite, which are at the core of this chapter, are an additional overlapping non-communicable condition of this non-infectious NTD.

Physiopathology of Snakebites

Snakes are predators that assault their prey through several different methods, including constriction, aggressive biting or envenomation. Even though they avoid human contact, snakebites can be enacted as defense, with bites more frequently involving the exposed extremities [1].

Snake venoms are encoded by genes that originally express proteins linked to various physiological functions. These multi-locus gene families generate extensive functional diversity while maintaining shared structural scaffolds [2]. Snake venoms typically consist of a mixture of 20 to more than 100 components, of which the majority (>90%) are peptides and proteins characterized by a range of bioactivities that can include neurotoxicity, haemotoxicity and cytotoxicity, depending on the snake species. Venom composition can vary widely between species and even within the same species, due to factors, such as environmental conditions [8]. Among the most important toxin classes, we can list phospholipases A2, snake venom metalloproteinases and snake venom serine proteases. In addition to the genetic determinants of venom, external factors such as diet influence toxin expression and overall venom composition [2]. Genetic and environmental factors lead to significant inter-specific and intra-specific variations in venom composition, as well as to geographical and seasonal variations [2].

Snakebites are always to be considered a medical emergency, because the complexity of snake venoms can cause an array of rapidly evolving, life-threatening and potentially disabling effects in victims [2]. This stated, not all bites by venomous snakes involve envenomation: "dry" bites occur in 2–50% of cases [1].

In cases where envenomation does occur, its related morbidity is characterized by several manifestations that can vary according to the snake species and the characteristics of its venom: among these, we can consider consumption coagulopathy, neurotoxicity with progressive paralysis or stroke [9–11], myotoxicity and compartment syndrome, cardiotoxicity and myocardial infarction or nephrotoxicity leading to acute or chronic renal failure [1]. Enzymes contained in the venom, like hyaluronidase and collagenase, proteinase or phospholipase can lead to local tissue injury and inflammation at the site of aggression, causing pain and oedema, which can extend from the site of the bite causing bullae and dermo necrosis [1].

Vessels can be involved in the physiopathology of snakebites in different ways. Lymphatic vessels have a double role in damage after snakebite; first, their involvement may contribute to the development and severity of the oedema and additionally, the venom can spread through them from the snakebite point to reach systemic circulation [1]. Enzymes like metalloproteinases can threaten the endothelial integrity, leading to microvascular damage and haemorrhage [1], potentially leading to macroscopic cardiovascular damage [12], which we will analyse in detail in the dedicated section. The pathophysiology of vascular damage in snakebites is summarized in Fig. 7.1.

Clinical Manifestations

When acquiring the patient's clinical history, it is important to collect information on the circumstances of the bite, including the time of day or night during which it occurred, the activity that the patient was performing during the attack and the environment surrounding the scene of the attack, all important details that could suggest what species of snake is more likely to be responsible of the aggression. In the absence of more specific clues, the species identity could be also inferred by specific clinical symptoms [2]. Evidence of envenoming is absent in 10–90% of bites by venomous snakes, which are known as dry bites, as observed earlier; in some other cases, symptoms may manifest only many hours after the bite. For this reason, snakebites are always considered a medical emergency, and patients who report a snakebite should be observed for at least 24 h [2].

Among the clinical manifestations, haemostatic disturbances are suggested by persistent bleeding from the fang punctures but spontaneous systemic bleeding distant from the bite site may occur, for example, mucosal bleeding, with the presence of blood in urine, sputum or stool. Cutaneous ecchymoses can also be present [2].

Signs of neurotoxicity include palpebral ptosis. In a later stage, descendent paralysis can be life-threatening, when it reaches the bulbar and respiratory muscles [2]. Hypovolaemia and hypovolemic shock can result from local extravasation of plasma or blood that can cause a massively swollen bitten limb. Shock can additionally be caused by myocardial damage due to venom effect on heart tissue or to coronary artery constriction, thrombosis or stress-induced hyper-catecholaminaemia [2].

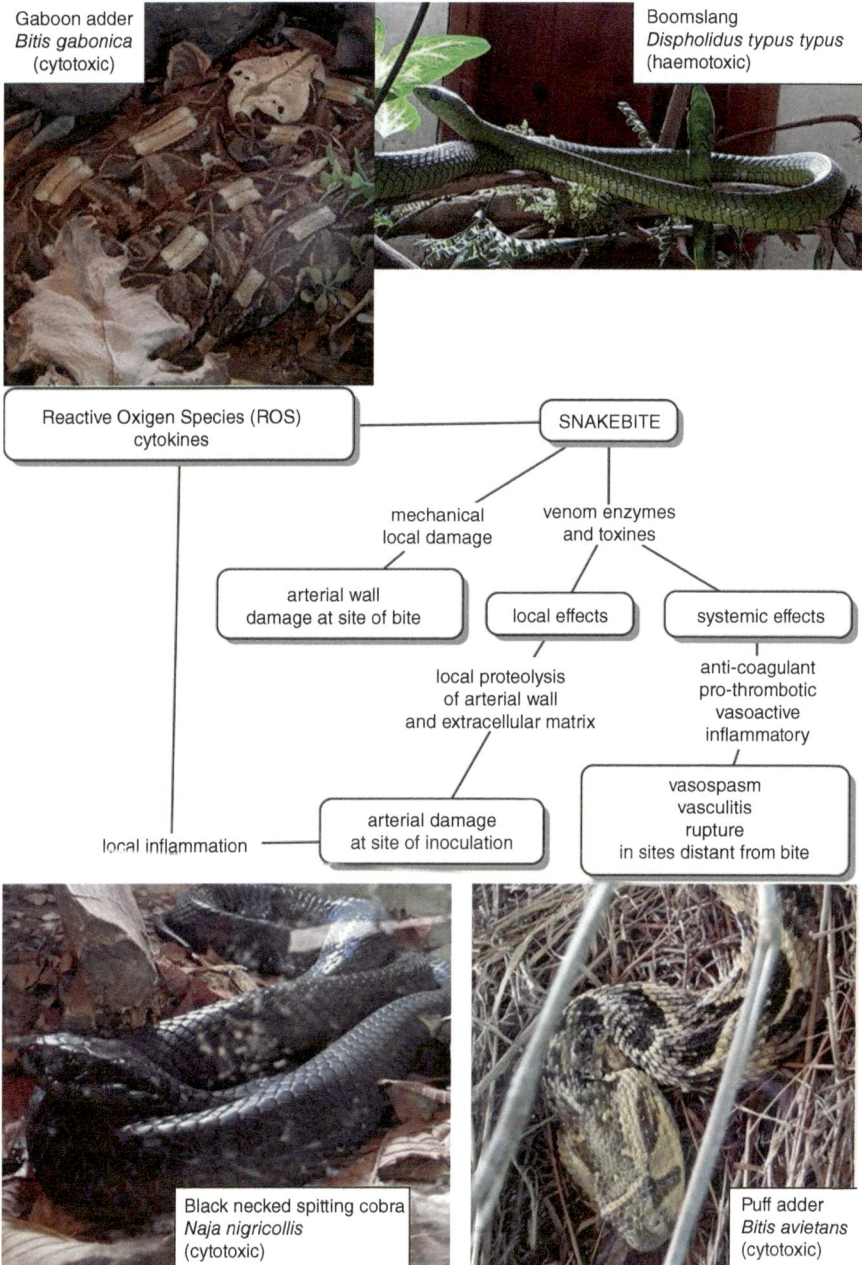

Fig. 7.1 Pathophysiology of vascular lesions in snakebites. Snakebites can cause vascular damage through local damage or through the local or systemic effect of venoms (cytolytic or haemotoxic). The photographs of snake species are original from the authors and were taken at Maserani snakepark, Arusha, Tanzania

Snakebite envenoming can lead to wound complications and also can have chronic effects on multiple organ systems, as occurs for the musculoskeletal apparatus or renal, endocrine and nervous systems. Notwithstanding the burden of these chronic issues, the chronic effects of envenomation are poorly understood, and cohort studies are rare [6]. As occurs for the delayed assessment in the acute phase after the envenomation, populations living in endemic low-middle income countries also face challenges in access to care and barriers to access to laboratory facilities and services to enable diagnosis of snakebite chronic sequelae; services and equipment and expertise are often unavailable in rural settings or can't be accessed due to financial constraints of survivors of snakebite. Misdiagnosis or delayed diagnosis of these chronic sequelae can impact survivors' quality of life [6]. As suggested for other NTDs, a system-oriented approach formed by multicomponent interventions to address chronic aspects of snakebite care, including social support programmes and incentives for multidisciplinary research, is needed [6].

Treatment of Snakebites

Treatment of snakebites can be divided into three phases: first of all basic physiologic functions must be preserved, through an urgent resuscitation and correction of respiratory circulatory and haemostatic failure. If signs of systemic envenoming become evident, the specific antivenom at an appropriate dosage must be promptly administered. Polyclonal antivenoms are, until now, the only clinically tested specific treatment for snakebite envenoming, produced by immunizing animals with selected snake venoms to stimulate the production of polyclonal neutralizing IgG antibodies [2]. This stage of medical management of anti-venom treatment is challenged by many different factors, including national procurement of inappropriate or ineffective antivenoms or the unavailability of functional cold chains [2]. Once envenoming is controlled by sub-ministration of appropriate anti-venom, addressing the issues that could lead to disability by early diagnosis and rehabilitation is essential to limit the morbidity in survivors [2]. A booster dose of tetanus toxoid is suggested in all snakebite cases [2].

Vascular Complications in Snakebite Envenomation

Vascular complications in victims of snakebites have been reported rarely in the literature, almost in isolated case reports or small monocentric experiences [13]. Our group retrieved through a review of literature (Medline, Scopus and Embase databases) the available published cases describing the clinical occurrence of peripheral and visceral arterial lesions after snakebite envenomation. As a search strategy, the used key words were "arterial lesions OR arterial rupture OR artery dissection OR arterial aneurysm AND snakebite". A summary of available evidences in literature, with cases published between 1982 and 2022, is reported in

Table 7.1 and contains anagraphic details, clinical presentation details, information on pharmacological and surgical management and outcome details that were available for each published case (Table 7.1).

The damage to the vascular system can be due to the direct lesion of the vessel at the bite site or to the effect of enzymes like metalloproteinases. Enzymes can threaten the endothelial integrity, leading to microvascular damage and haemorrhage [1] or to macroscopic cardiovascular damage [12].

The damaged arteries can be of both peripheral and visceral districts, with clinical manifestations occurring soon after aggression but also after days from the bite. It is important to keep in mind that rarely reported complications of snakebites, as in the case of vascular lesions, can occur from days to weeks after envenomation, due to enzymatic components of venom or to the mechanical injury at the bite site [13]. Even though signs of local damage can be present in patients with vascular damage, it is also important to consider that vascular lesions are occasionally reported in patients in the absence of local effects [13]. Senthilkumaran et al. have suggested that arterial damage in the absence of surrounding tissue involvement could occur in cases in which intra-arterial injection of the venom occurred through wall penetration [13] or because of the local action of the venom injected in proximity of the involved artery [13, 14].

Direct Arterial Damage

Damage to the arteries can be direct and manifest at the site of bite, immediately as a result of trauma or in the following days. Lesions may consist of pseudo-aneurysms in the arteries located in the districts that are the site of the bite. Senthilkumaran et al. have described two cases of pseudo-aneurysms after a bite in the antecubital fossa, which occurred as pulsatile masses in correspondence with the ulnar artery some days after the attack [15]. The direct damage to the artery also occurred in the case of a radial artery aneurysm occurring after a snakebite in the proximity of the hand [14]. These lesions occurring in sites exposed to bites, usually limbs, may also be prone to overlap of compartment syndrome, as in the case of radial aneurysm described by Linfeng et al. [14].

Damage Mediated by Venom Enzymes

The arterial damage can be mediated by a proteolytic enzymatic component of the venom (metalloproteinase, serine proteases or phospholipase A2), which can destroy the structural components of the arterial wall or its extracellular matrix or through the direct endothelial damage, with the induction of apoptosis in endothelial cells [13, 15]. In addition, enzymes can cause the necrosis of arterial walls and surrounding tissues [14], or they can activate inflammatory mechanisms mediated by reactive oxygen species and cytokines, leading to inflammatory damage of

Table 7.1 Summary of snakebite case reports retrieved from literature

	Author/year	Age	Sex	Geographic location	location of bite	Arterial segment involved	Clinical manifestation	Treatment	Aneurysm treatment	Outcome
1	Senthilkumaran 2022	22	M	India	Ankle	Inferior renal polar artery (rupture)	Severe local pain, swelling, gum bleeding At 36 hours: haematuria, conjunctival haemorrhage At 72 h: severe diffused abdominal pain, vomit At 76 h: hypotension, renal insufficiency	80 mL polyvalent antivenom[a] 36 h additional 200 mg antivenom	Emergency selective coil angioembolisation (inferior pole renal artery)	ALIVE Month 3: complete resolution of the haematoma - Normal-sized right kidney
2	Senthilkumaran 2022	50	F	India	Left cubital fossa	Ulnar artery pseudo-aneurysm	Day 4: 4 cm cubital mass with thrill. Normal distal flow No signs of local or systemic envenomation	On emergency access 200 mL of polyvalent antivenom[a]	Ultrasound guided compression of pseudo-aneurysm (day 4–5–6)	ALIVE Week 2: reduction in aneurysm size, patent artery, no functional impairment
3	Senthilkumaran 2022	45	F	India	Right cubital fossa	Ulnar artery pseudo-aneurysm (antecubital fossa)	2 h: resolution of coagulopathy with antivenom Day 5: swelling at bite site; Day 6: hand paraesthesia, pain 1 week 3 cm pulsatile mass	2 h after bite: 250 mL of polyvalent antivenom	Ultrasound-guided compression of pseudo-aneurysm and thrombin injection (day4–5–6)	ALIVE Week 2: reduction aneurysm size, patent artery, no functional impairment

(continued)

4	Linfeng 2020	65	M	China	Hand	Radial artery aneurysm	10 h: local swelling, pain, forearm-paraesthesia 17 h: Compartment syndrome	3 h after bite: 8000 units of anti-venom (anti-*Deinagkistrodon acutus*) dexamethasone, 20% mannitol, furosemide	Back palm incisions Day 3 radial aneurysmectomy Day 17 artery and vein reconstruction, femoral skin flap graft; 20 h post-surgery: Graft failure and hand ischemia	ALIVE LIMB LOSS Day 18: Major limb amputation (ischemia)
5	Lee 2019	62	M	Korea		Splenic artery bleeding	Day 3: dizziness and loss of consciousness. Intermittent hypotension. Sudden abdominal pain.	At bite: antivenom At surgery: packed red blood cells and Agkistrodon antivenom 6000 U) for 3 days	Splenic-artery embolization	ALIVE Day 4 CT scan: successful embolization, hemoperitoneum reduction
6	Malbranque 2008	74	M	Martinique	Left elbow	Intramural cardiac vessels dissection	Day 2: limb swelling unconsciousness, tetraplegia cerebral infarcts, myocardial infarction patent coronaries Day 6: atrial fibrillation, left ventricular failure, mitral valve rupture	Day 2 after bite: Specific antivenom therapy (80 mL of Bothrofav e.v.)	Exitus before treatment	EXITUS Day 10 after bite: cardiogenic shock, myocardial infarction and rupture of papillary muscle of mitral valve

(continued)

Table 7.1 (continued)

	Author/year	Age	Sex	Geographic location	location of bite	Arterial segment involved	Clinical manifestation	Treatment	Aneurysm treatment	Outcome
7	Ahn 2007	82	F	Korea	Index finger	Hepatic artery-distal branches haemorrhage	Day 4 after bite: hypotension, coagulopathy, anaemia, abdominal pain and distension	Conservative treatment of the bite	Hepatic artery embolization (4th or 5th ordered branch hepatic arteries and inferior phrenic artery	ALIVE 2 weeks after embolization drainage of post-haemorrhagic liver pseudocyst Week 16: decreased cyst volume
8	Jonas 1982	na	na	Germany	na	Posterior-tibial artery pseudoaneurysm	na	na	na	na

[a]Polyvalent antivenom 'Big Four'snakes [Russell' viper, cobra (Naja naja), krait (Bungarus caeruleus) and saw-scaled viper(Echis carinatus)] of India (Bharat Serums and Vaccines, India)

M male, *F* female, *n.a.* not-available, *e.v.* endovenous

arteries and tissues [13]. The direct effect of venom on the target vessel can affect micro-vessels, causing severe vasospasm and toxic vasculitis, finally leading to artery rupture and focal leakage [16]. Pre-existent defects in the arterial districts can predispose vessels to further injury after the exposure to venom toxins [15].

Compartment Syndrome

In addition to the direct damage induced by the bite or by the effect of venom enzymes on the vascular structures, compartment syndrome is also described as a clinical manifestation of vascular interest potentially occurring after snakebite or as a consequence of its popular management through the use of tourniquet.

Compartment syndrome can occur when envenoming occurs in muscles contained in tight fascial compartments, such as the anterior tibial compartment. Envenomation and trauma leading to sufficient swelling can compromise blood supply to the limb [2]. In addition to the effect of the venom, some popular practices enacted to attempt treatment could increase the risk of compartment syndrome in the attempt to self-manage the snakebite. Among these local remedies, one that represents a significant threat to the vascular prognosis of affected limbs is the popular use of a tourniquet. A recent study from Tanzania has listed tourniquets, the local incision at the bite site and the application of a snake stone as popular remedies, used by more than 80% of the victims before seeking hospital treatment [17].

On assessment, when compartment syndrome develops, the affected limbs may appear painful, tender, tensely swollen, cold, cyanosed and pulseless, manifesting classic clinical signs that call for surgical decompression through fasciotomy [2]. Some differences in compartment syndrome secondary to snakebites have been described when compared to other aetiologies of this syndrome. One of these differences is the fact that the results of the direct measurements of intra-compartmental pressure are usually normal in limbs affected by snakebite, rejecting a classical diagnosis of compartment syndrome. On the other side, experimental evidence suggests that muscles sufficiently envenomed to cause a sustained increase in intra-compartmental pressure are usually not viable and may not benefit from fasciotomy [2], making surgical management challenging. As a complication of vascular interest, compartment syndrome after snakebite also contributes to the outcome of limb loss [14].

Arterial Damage and Anti-venom Administration

A prompt anti-venom administration as soon as envenomation clinical signs appear is essential to limit the clinical consequences in snakebite victims. Severe clinical manifestations such as haemoperitoneum due to visceral artery bleeding or myocardial infarction due to intramural cardiac vessels dissection [12, 16] were reported in patients not receiving anti-venom treatment after snakebite.

But we should also consider that arterial damage was described in some cases notwithstanding prompt anti-venom treatment [18] or after an initial positive response to it [13]. It was suggested in previous reports that because the total venom load is usually unknown, the initial anti-venom dose selected to arrest or reverse the immediate effects of the venom could be insufficient, and delayed complications may still occur if the dosage is not adjusted to the clinical response in the hours following the first dose [1].

The reasons behind missed or mistreatment that contribute to challenging the clinical outcome of these patients could be the seeking of local remedies rather than hospital assessment and treatment [19, 20]. The use of traditional remedies can be due to cultural beliefs, financial issues for long travel distances and hospitalization and lack of anti-venom at healthcare facilities [17, 19–21]. The diffused use of tourniquet application as self-remedy before reaching the health facility could favour the occurrence of this complication and should be discouraged [20], and these issues should be considered and addressed by stakeholders and policymakers.

Diagnostic and Surgical Management

Ultrasound assessment of arterial damage has been suggested as a reliable diagnostic tool in the case of suspected arterial damage after a snake bite [13, 14].

Ultrasound-guided compression of the pseudoaneurysm, when feasible, has been described as effective as a non-invasive approach to pseudo-aneurysm peripheral lesions, leading to resolution with or without the additional aid of prothrombin injection to help pseudo-aneurysm sac thrombosis [13].

In some settings, especially when visceral involvement is suspected, additional diagnostic tools such as CT or angiography scans may be of help in visualizing organ damage and the site of bleeding [15, 16, 18]. In the case of an angiographic approach to the diagnosis of visceral bleeding, especially in those cases where small distal branches are responsible for internal haemorrhage, selective endovascular embolization was suggested as an effective treatment, as reported by Ahn et al. in a case of hepatic artery distal branch rupture with haemoperitoneum, treated by embolization with coils and gelatine sponge sheet [16] or in a case of splenic artery bleeding reported by Lee [18] or of the inferior polar renal artery in the case of Wunderlich syndrome reported by Senthilkumaran [15].

Compartment syndrome has to be considered and promptly treated in snakebite victims to prevent limb ischemia and limb loss [22]. In cases in which compartment syndrome occurs, fasciotomy can be considered, but with caution. Compartment syndrome in victims of snake envenomation may differ clinically from compartment syndrome secondary to different aetiology, as analysed in the previous chapter. Fasciotomy is challenging in these cases not only because it could prove to be ineffective, in case of massive envenomation, to improve the limb prognosis, but also because of the surgical risk in cases with concomitant haemostatic impairment, if surgery is performed before the restoration of a normal coagulation by anti-venom administration [2]. Even in cases successfully managed with fasciotomy, international experts have emphasized that because this intervention can also cause permanent morbidity and increase hospital stay, fasciotomy for people bitten by a snake should be discouraged and reserved for the treatment of complicating necrotizing bacterial fasciitis or myositis [2].

The post-operatory follow-up to exclude coagulopathy or rebleeding is highly recommended to confirm the resolution of the lesion, assess response to treatment and improve patient outcomes [18].

The necrotizing effects of venom could lead to complications after surgery, as reported by Linfeng, where aneurysmectomy and skin graft were complicated by thrombosis of the reconstructed vasculature and by skin graft failure, leading to ischaemia requiring superior limb amputation [14]. Compartment syndrome complicated the arterial reconstruction in this case, contributing to the outcome of limb loss [14].

Management of lesions should finally take into consideration the specific local physiopathology and avoid treatments that could additionally impair tissue repair during the management of snakebite wounds, like a high concentration of hydrogen peroxide, large doses of steroids and diuretics [22].

Conclusions and Recommendations

The severity of clinical manifestations, the morbidity and the frequently associated life-threatening challenges that come along with vascular damage call for the need to inquire better about the occurrence of vessel damage in snakebite injuries. Missed and mistreatment, which can occur due to the lack of tools, drug storage, and appropriate training of healthcare workers, should be prevented with further research and interventions that could address the local needs [20]. Challenges when seeking treatment include recognizing venomous snakes, giving first aid and reaching a healthcare centre that has anti-venom and trained personnel available, barriers that have to be addressed to provide adequate care to snakebite victims [21].

In this perspective, the implementation of programmes aiming at the reduction of snakebite envenomation fatalities by WHO is a relatively recent reality. This includes a systematic report of cases that should include the specific challenge of cardiovascular morbidity and herpetological speciation according to an area of interest and venom characterization, to achieve data that could better guide the clinical practice and the policies in the future.

Considering the WHO's goal to halve the number of snakebite-related deaths and disabilities by 2030 through preventive efforts, improved treatments and enhanced access to care [1], studies focusing on specific aspects of this neglected tropical condition are needed to guide future investigations.

Acknowledgements The authors are thankful to Prof. Tito Lanoi, Herpetologist at College of African Wildlife Mangement, for the precious inputs from his professional experience in Tanzania, which guided the focus on hot topics to be emphasized in this chapter.

The chapter covers a topic that was presented in the form of abstract during the fourth NCD Scientific Conference, in Mwanza, 10–11 November 2022.

The authors are thankful to the contributors to this previous work, specifically Pankras Luoga, Mwanahawa Mshana and Hoseenu Palilo, from the Department of Parasitology and Medical Entomology, Muhimbili University of Health and Applied Science, Dar es Salaam, Tanzania; Witness M. Bonaventura, from the Kilimanjaro Christian Medical University College, Tanzania; Nyanda C. Justine, from the Department of Medical Parasitology and Entomology, Catholic University of Health and Allied Sciences, Mwanza, Tanzania; Yonah Yangaza, Muhimbi University of Heath and Allied Science, Dar es Salaam, Tanzania, Nathanael Ndagiwe, Tumbi regional referral hospital, Coastal region in Tanzania.

References

1. Seifert SA, Armitage JO, Sanchez EE. Snake envenomation. N Engl J Med. 2022;386(1):68–78.
2. Warrell DA, Williams DJ. Clinical aspects of snakebite envenoming and its treatment in low-resource settings. Lancet. 2023;401(10385):1382–98. https://doi.org/10.1016/S0140-6736(23)00002-8.
3. Golding W. The Brooklyn papyrus snakebite and medicinal treatments' Magico-religious context. Religions. 2023;14(1300)
4. Ana MR. Toxicology and snakes in ptolemaic Egyptian dynasty: the suicide of Cleopatra. Toxicol Rep. 2021;8:676–95. https://doi.org/10.1016/j.toxrep.2021.03.004.
5. Zacharia F, Silvestri V, Mushi V, Ogweno G, Makene T, Mhamilawa LE. Burden and factors associated with ongoing transmission of soil-transmitted helminths infections among the adult population: a community-based cross-sectional survey in Muleba district, Tanzania. PLoS One. 2023;18(7):e0288936. https://doi.org/10.1371/journal.pone.0288936.
6. Bhaumik S, Gopalakrishnan M, Meena P. Mitigating the chronic burden of snakebite: turning the tide for survivors. Lancet. 2021;398(10309):1389–90. https://doi.org/10.1016/S0140-6736(21)01905-X.
7. Abouyannis M, Esmail H, Hamaluba M, Ngama M, Mwangudzah H, Mumba N, et al. A global core outcome measurement set for snakebite clinical trials. Lancet Glob Heal. 2023;11(2):e296–300.
8. Oliveira AL, Viegas MF, da Silva SL, Soares AM, Ramos MJ, Fernandes PA. The chemistry of snake venom and its medicinal potential. Nat Rev Chem. 2022;6(7):451–69.
9. Ozen S, Guzel S. A case of ischaemic stroke following cerastes cerastes snake bite in Libya. Afr J Neurol Sci. 2020;39(1):21–4.
10. Chani M, Abouzahir A, Haimeur C, Kamili ND, Mion G. Accident vasculaire cerebral ischemique a` la suite d'une envenimation viperine grave au Maroc, traitee par un antivenin inadapte. Ann Fr Anesth Reanim. 2012;31:82–5.
11. Dabilgou AA, Sondo A, Dravé A, Diallo I, Marie J, Kyelem A, et al. Hemorrhagic stroke following snake bite in Burkina Faso (West Africa). A case series. Trop Dis Travel Med Vaccines. 2021;6:1–6.
12. Malbranque S, Piercecchi-marti MD, Thomas L, Barbey C, Courcier D, Bucher B, et al. Case report: fatal diffuse thrombotic microangiopathy after a bite by the " Fer-de-Lance" pit viper (Bothrops lanceolatus) of Martinique. Am J Trop Med Hyg. 2008;78(6):856–61.
13. Russell C, Senthilkumaran S, Miller SW, Williams HF, Vaiyapuri R, Savania R, et al. Ultrasound-guided compression method effectively counteracts Russell's viper bite-induced pseudoaneurysm. Toxins. 2022;14(4):4–11.
14. Linfeng W, Lutao X, Pin L, Linjie L, Meisong C, Wang D. Toxicon radial artery aneurysm formation and spontaneous rupture after snake bite to the right forearm. Toxicon. 2020;181(April):79–81.

15. Senthilkumaran S, Miller SW, Williams HF, Savania R, Thirumalaikolundusubramanian P, Patel K, et al. Toxicon development of Wunderlich syndrome following a Russell' s viper bite. Toxicon. 2022;215:11–6.

16. Ahn JH, Choi S, Lee JH, Park MS. Hemoperitoneum caused by hepatic necrosis and rupture following a snakebite: a case report with rare CT findings and successful embolization. 2007;8(December):556–60.

17. Id SI, Justin J, Hamasaki K, Konje ET, Kongola GW. Assessment of snakebite management practices at Meserani Juu in Monduli District, Northern Tanzania. PLoS One. 2022;7:1–12.

18. Lee HS. A case of non-operative management of atraumatic splenic hemorrhage due to snakebite venom-induced consumption coagulopathy. Am J Case Rep. 2019:1314–9.

19. Patikorn C, Ismail AK, Asnawi S, Abidin Z, Blanco FB, Blessmann J, et al. Situation of snakebite, antivenom market and access to antivenoms in ASEAN countries. BMJ Glob Heal 2022;7(3):1–11.

20. Margono F, Outwater AH, Wilson ML, Howell KM. Bärnighausen T, Snakebite treatment in tanzania: identifying gaps in community practices and hospital resources. Int J Environ Res Public Health. 2022:1–14.

21. NMCP. The United Republic of Tanzania National guidelines for malaria diagnosis, treatment and preventive therapies 2020.

22. Cheng C, Chiang L, Ho C, Liu P, Lai K, Lin W, et al. Ulnar artery pseudoaneurysm and compartment syndrome formation after snake bite to the left forearm by Lan Pin et al. Clin Toxicol. 2017;20(17):1–2.

Conclusions

8

Contents

The General Rise in Vascular Non-communicable Diseases in LMIC

The aim of this book was to investigate on "the neglected area of vascular surgery", targeting vascular pathology in the context of neglected populations, in countries with low resources, low access to medical and surgical care and in concomitance with historically neglected endemic diseases. As emphasized in the introduction to this book, vascular damage in patients affected by NTDs could follow patterns that are different from the one occurring in classic atherosclerosis, and the understanding of the pathophysiology behind vascular lesions in this specific clinical setting, of their clinical manifestations and of their natural course is urgently needed. This knowledge will constitute an essential tool to target comorbidity management, and to design prevention and control interventions aiming at lowering and interrupting disease transmission and morbidity burden, as indicated in the new WHO roadmap.

The neglect towards vascular surgery as a discipline in low- and middle-income countries (LMICs) is not limited to the multi-disciplinary issues that are at the heart of this book. It is, on the contrary, a part of a wider gap in knowledge and practice that transversally involves all areas of surgery as a discipline, from pathophysiology to epidemiology to diagnostics and treatment options, and as such it should be addressed in future research.

Non-communicable diseases (NCDs) represent a major public health concern globally, rapidly increasing in prevalence in LMICs. The World Health Organization estimated that these conditions are responsible each year for 71% of deaths globally, quantifyable as 41 million deaths yearly, 74% of which occurring in low-resources settings. In regions with resources shortage, the majority of premature deaths (86%) also occur. Trying to figure out a future scenario, it was suggested that, for 2030, around 80% of NCDs attributable deaths will come from LMICs, predicting about 52 million deaths yearly [1].

Analysing the epidemiology of NCDs according to the type of cardiovascular manifestations in lower-income countries, aortic aneurysm, ischaemic stroke and peripheral artery disease accounted for 2.2% of deaths and 0.8% of DALYs [2]. During the past decade, an increase in mortality attributable to these main vascular conditions was reported. The number of deaths per 100,000 people due to aortic aneurysm from 1990 to 2019 increased by 100% and 60% in upper-middle and lower-income countries, respectively [2]. Also for peripheral artery diseases, lower-middle-income countries and low-income countries saw an increase of 60% and 28% in mortality, with an increased DALY of 67% and 60%, respectively [2].

Vascular Surgery: Challenges in Low- and Middle-Income Countries

In order to address the issue of NDCs in LMICs, we need to address those challenges that are related to this specific setting, as the insufficient availability of quality diagnostic tools; the barriers impairing the access of patients to quality surgery; the challenges in the research system, including the lack of available data. The awareness of the fact that vascular surgery in LMIC needs to operate in a peculiar scenario which is very different from where the core knowledge of this discipline was built is crucial . The need to re-analyse vascular surgery from research to implementation faces several barriers, which were analysed in a very interesting state-of-the-art review recently published by Bencheikh et al. [2].

Impaired Access to Treatment

According to this review, one of the major challenges faced by LMICs in addressing the vascular surgery conditions is that the increased need of care emphasized by recent epidemiological data is still not translated into an increased access to treatment. The insufficient number of available specialists is one of the barriers to provision of treatment. In countries like Ethiopia, the access to vascular surgery services is very low, with 0.25 vascular surgeons per 10 million people, which is 27,400 times less than that in the United States [2].

The lack of suitable infrastructure including operating theatres, frequent power outages and inadequate surgical equipment and supplies are an additional barrier. The lack of access to advanced diagnostic and therapeutic tools (like computed tomography angiography, angiography suit, reliable electricity and endovascular tools) obstacolate the instalment of vascular survices in LMICs [2].

Lack of Data Registries and Involvement in Surgery International Networks

Another important factor, which is a consequence of the unavailability of suitable and safely managed informatic infrastructures and qualified personnel to collect information, is the lack of data recording systems from LMICs. While international registries are used to share data that can guide practice, leading to important international collaborations, LMICs are scarcely represented in these networks [2]. Data are essential in describing the epidemiology of health conditions in endemic settings, and the lack of access to reliable disease data archives is one of the major challenges that affect the ability to address unique clinical problems related to developing countries and limits global researchers' ability to learn from diverse populations [3]. Despite the introduction of electronic health data systems in LMIC to improve the availability, quantity and quality of data, many countries were left behind [3]. These data sets would be essential also to understand the prevalence, clinical presentation, natural history and outcome of specific comorbidities related to NTD, which up until now have been described only in occasional case reports or series. Retrospective database could expand the number and quality of observations needed to define the hypothesis, guiding future research in unexplored patterns.

Speciality Training

The lack of infrastructures, of data registries and of the representation of LMICs in global vascular surgery networks also negatively impacts on the training on vascular surgeons, with limited opportunities for formation that certainly don't meet the increasing demand for professionals [2]. At the level of speciality training, courses are not standardized and are usually included in the general surgery programmes. Additionally, the unique disease burden intersecting with vascular disease in these countries, like the diseases described in this book, but also others such as HIV and Buerger's disease necessitate specific training to best intervene in this setting [2].

Financial Issues

Another fact that we should not ignore when analysing barriers to the development of vascular surgery services in low -resources settings is that vascular surgery is a highly specialized branch of surgery that carries high cost, and this cost would impact at individual, family and national healthcare level [2]. Endovascular services carry an additional cost, and the policy for insurance to cover these expenses is actually different for LMICs, constituting an enormous barrier to treatment [2]. There is an urgent need to allow the effective delivery of these diagnostic and interventional tools and to reduce medical costs for the management of surgical vascular diseases in this setting, in order to improve the quality of life among affected populations: enhancing access to essential medicines and basic technologies is crucial for the accomplishment of the Millennium Development Goals [1], and these goals should be consolidated at implementational level.

Education Issues on Vascular Surgery Matters

Finally, challenges are also eradicated at a population level. Knowledge and beliefs related to vascular surgery issues among the population can impact on access to services. Mistrust for the healthcare system can reduce the access to treatment and seeking care, and the improvement of knowledge of vascular disease could change this trend in this setting.

The challenges faced by LMICs in the institution of vascular surgery services are summarized in Fig. 8.1.

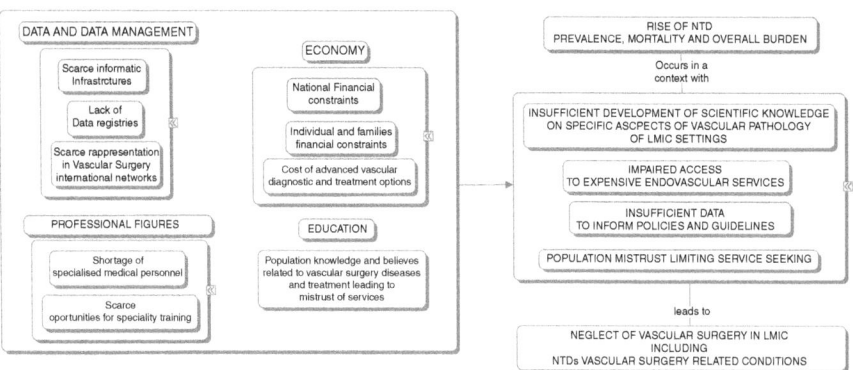

Fig. 8.1 Vascular surgery: challenges in LMICs

Future Research

This book was based mainly on available evidences in literature from cases and case series related to vascular issues of surgical interest in patients affected by NTDs. These narrow evidences were summarized to provide a general view on this multidisciplinary topic. We believe in its value as an input to inspire further research.

First of all, we believe that the increase in reports and case series related to these topics will be crucial in the immediate future to ignite the dialogue on the topic and to better focus on emerging gaps that need to be addressed more urgently. Case reports are the lower level of evidence, but at this stage of investigation on the neglected aspects of vascular issues in NTDs can be determinant to define research questions that need to be answered. In addition, case reports are a valuable teaching tool in the academic environment and could be an important link between theory, clinical practice and research in the academic environment in countries endemic for NTDs.

The institution of data registries in endemic countries and the participation in international data sharing networks will be essential in the next years not only to address the specific vascular burden related to NTD in endemic countries but also to inform the clinical practice in non-endemic settings. The morbidity of vascular surgical interest related to NTDs can be chronic and can occur many years after infection. The increase in populations movements due to international travel, displacement and emigration will increase the number of cases that will reach full clinical attention in non-endemic settings, with the consequent need for clinicians to be prepared on these previously exceptional clinical issues.

The new WHO's comprehensive multidisciplinary perspective of addressing NTDs [4, 5], which includes a transversal approach to different diseases and from a multidisciplinary perspective, is essential to fully understand also the cardiovascular epidemiology in endemic regions of the world and how neglected conditions impact on clinical features and outcome among endemic populations.

The journey to bring a full access to vascular theatre for a full management of surgical vascular diseases, to address the increasing, in some way specific and complex need among the populations which were left behind in the incredible progress of our discipline in the last decades, will be tough and will have to cover all aspects of Surgery, from surgical research to ethical debate.

References

1. Albelbeisi AH, Albelbeisi A, El Bilbeisi AH, Taleb M, Takian A, Akbari-Sari A. Public sector capacity to prevent and control of noncommunicable diseases in twelve low- and middle-income countries based on WHO-PEN standards: a systematic review. Heal Serv Insights. 2021;14:1178632920986233.
2. Bencheikh N, Zarrintan S, Quatramoni JG, Al-Nouri O, Malas M, Gaffey AC. Vascular surgery in low-income and middle-income countries: a state-of-the-art review. Ann Vasc Surg. 2023;95:297–306. https://doi.org/10.1016/j.avsg.2023.05.024.

3. Abdul-rahman T, Ghosh S, Lukman L, Bamigbade GB, Oladipo OV, Amarachi OR, et al. Income countries: mystery behind public health statistics and measures. J Infect Public Health. 2023;16(10):1556–61. https://doi.org/10.1016/j.jiph.2023.07.001.
4. WHO. Ending the neglect to attain the sustainable development goals: a road map for neglected tropical diseases 2021–2030. WHO; 2020. 196 p.
5. Ending the neglect to attain the Sustainable Development Goals: a strategic framework for integrated control and management of skin-related neglected tropical diseases. Geneva: World Health Organization; 2022. Available at: https://www.who.int/publications/i/item/9789240010352.

Index